THERAPEUTICS OF TUBERCULOSIS

(PULMONARY CONSUMPTION)

WM. H. BURT. M.D.
OF CHICAGO, ILLINOIS

AUTHOR OF "CHARACTERISTIC MATERIA MEDICA," A MONOGRAPH ON
"POLYPORUS OFFICINALIS, POLYPORUS PINICOLA, USTILAGO
MAYDIS, AND CHINCHONA OFFICINALIS."

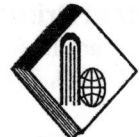

B. Jain Publishers (P) Ltd.
New Delhi

Note

Any information given in this book is not intended to be taken as a replacement for medical advice. Any person with a condition requiring medical attention should consult a qualified practitioner or therapist.

Reprint edition : 2006

All right are reserved. No part of this publication may be reproduced, stored in a retrieval system or transmitted, in any form or by any means, mechanical, recording or otherwise, without prior written permission of the publishers

Price. Rs. 79.00

© Copyright with the Publisher

Published by :
Kuldeep Jain
For
B. Jain Publishers (P.) Ltd.
1921, Street No.10, Chuna Mandi
Paharganj, New Delhi-110 055 (INDIA)
Phones: 91-011-2358 0800, 2358 1100, 2358 1300
Fax: 91-011-2358 0471; *Email:* bjain@vsnl.com
Website: www.bjainbooks.com

Printed in India by
J.J. Offset Printers
522, FIE, Patpar Ganj, Delhi - 110 092
Phones: 2216 9633, 2215 6128

ISBN : 81-7021-988-4
BOOK CODE : BB-5437

To

JOHN MEYHOFFER, M.D.

OF

NICE,

IN CONSIDERATION OF THE GREAT BENEFIT DERIVED FROM YOUR LABORS
FOUND IN YOUR TREATISE ON CHRONIC DISEASES OF THE ORGANS
OF RESPIRATION, I WOULD MOST RESPECTFULLY DEDICATE
TO YOU THIS, MY HUMBLE EFFORT, WITH GRATITUDE.

THE AUTHOR

Contents

	Page Nos.
INTRODUCTORY	(1)
MEDICAL TREATMENT	(4)
GENERAL ATONIC CONDITION OF THE BODY	(11)
EMACIATION AND DEBILITY	(18)
HÆMOPTYSIS	(46)
COUGH	(63)
ASTHMA	(166)
HECTIC FEVER AND NIGHT SWEATS	(220)
APHTHAE	(231)
DIARRHEA	(238)
PAIN	(240)
BED SORES	(242)
SPIROMETER	(246)

INTRODUCTORY

TUBERCULOSIS OR PULMONARY CONSUMPTION

It is estimated that more than one-eighth of the entire mortality of the human family is due to the fatal ravages of *tuberculosis*. It is, therefore, not only the most frequent of constitutional, but also the most common of all diseases. With these facts before the physician, it behoves him to make it's treatment a life study.

Tuberculous matter is an unorganized material, characterized by a soft, cheesy, pale or yellowish gray coloured substance deposited into all the organs and tissues of the body, *especially* the *lungs,* accompanied by persistent cough, expectoration of mucus, blood and pus, dyspnea, asthma, hectic fever, emaciation, night sweats, apthae, diarrhea, pain, bed sores, general atonic condition of the body and debility.

In persuing the works of various authors who have written elaborately upon the pathology and treatment of this dreaded disease, the writer's attention was directed to the catalogue of *distinct characteristic symptoms* of pulmonary tuberculosis, each of which presented itself as a subject for profitable study. Impressed with this idea, we have divided pulmonary tuberculosis into twelve of it's most prominent characteristic symptoms, and given a plenary treatment of each symptom by it self, believing that in doing so it would greatly aid the practitioner in successfully combating it's fatal ravages. They are the following:

1. General atonic condition of the body.
2. Emaciation.
3. Debility.
4. Haemoptysis.
5. Cough.
6. Asthma.
7. Hectic fever.
8. Night sweats.
9. Aphthae.
10. Diarrhea.
11. Pain.
12. Bed sores.

The pathology of the disease has been entirely omitted, it being so fully written up in our works on pathology, which are in the hands of every practitioner.

In writing the treatment of each symptom, we have collected together from our text books and journals all that has been written on this disease, and put in such shape that the busy physician and student can grasp and utilize it at once, without having to search over his whole library whenever a case presents itself for treatment.

The remedies have been so fully written, that not only the general indications are complete, but a *Characteristic Materia Medica* has been produced that forms a marked feature of the work, and we believe will be prized by the profession as invaluable; in it, the *heart* and *soul* of each remedy is put in such a concise shape that the labor of applying it to disease is made easy.

INTRODUCTORY

We have aimed to put nothing in this work but actual *practical, clinical experience,* something that can be turned to by the student with the feeling that what he is wielding has been *thoroughly tested* and *found reliable.*

MEDICAL TREATMENT

Before giving the indications for our remedies, it will not only be interesting, but practical, to note down the remedies used in our standard works for this formidable disease.

Dr. B. Baehr, in his "Science of Therapeutics" uses forty remedies, namely:

Aconite,	Cannabis,	Kali carb.,	Pulsatilla,
Alumina,	China,	Kali nit.,	Plumbum,
Arnica,	Cuprum,	Kreosote,	Phos. acid,
Belladonna,	Causticum,	Ledum,	Spongia,
Bryonia,	Cod liver oil,	Lycopodium,	Stannum,
Bromine,	Digitalis,	Manganum,	Silicea,
Baryta carb.,	Ferrum,	Millefolium,	Sulphur,
Calc. carb.,	Hepar sulph.,	Morphine,	Tartar emetic,
Calc. phos.,	Ipecac,	Natrium m.,	Veratrum alb.
Carbo veg.,	Iodine,	Phosphorus,	

Dr. W. Hitchman, in his work on consumption gives us forty eight remedies, namely:

Aconite,	Conium,	Hepar sulph.,	Pulsatilla,
Arsenicum,	Chelidonium,	Ipecac,	Plumbum,
Arnica,	Chinin. sulph.,	Iodine,	Phosphorus,
Ant. crud.,	Coffea,	Kali iod.,	Phos. acid,
Acid sulph.,	Cocculus,	Kali bi.,	Rheum,
Argentum,	Chamomilla,	Lachesis,	Sulphur,

MEDICAL TREATMENT

Acid nit.,	Camphor,	Laurocerasus,	Petroleum,
Belladonna,	Cuprum,	Lamium,	Terebinth.,
Bryonia,	Digitalis,	Merc. cor.,	Tartar emetic,
China,	Elaps,	Nux vom.,	Veratrum alb.,
Cannabis,	Ferrum,	Opium,	Zincum.
Cantharis,	Gamboge,	Oleum ricini,	

Dr. C. H. G. Jahr, in his "Forty Years Practice," gives thirty three remedies, but he doubts the virtues of the last ten, as indicated in his work:

Aconite,	Ferrum,	Lachesis,	Rhus tox.,
Bromine,	Hepar sulph.,	Mercury,	Sulphur,
Belladonna,	Iodine,	Nux vom.,	Spongia,
Bryonia,	Ipecac,	Nitric acid,	Silicea,
Calc. carb.,	Kali carb.,	Phos. acid,	Stannum,
Carbo veg.,	Kali iod.,	Phosphorus,	Sambucus.
China,	Kreosote,	Plumbum,	
Drosera,	Ledum,	Psorinum,	
Dulcamara,	Lycopodium,	Pulsatilla,	

Dr. C.G. Raue, in his "Practice," gives twenty six remedies:

Aconite,	Dulcamara,	Lycopodium,	Spongia,
Apis mel.,	Ferrum,	Myrtus communis,	Stannum,
Arsenicum,	Gelsemium,	Nitric acid,	Sulphur,
Carbo veg.,	Hepar sulph.,	Opium,	Tartar emetic,
Calc. carb.,	Iodine,	Phosphorus,	Veratrum alb.
China,	Kali carb.,	Sanguinaria,	
Cimicifuga,	Lachesis,	Silicea,	

Drs. Marcy and Hunt, in their work on "Practice," give thirty five remedies, viz:

Aconite,	Cod liver oil,	Ipecac,	Phos. acid,
Arnica,	Cuprum,	Iodium,	Phosphorus,

Alcohol,	China,	Kali iod.,	Sambucus,
Amm. carb.,	Digitalis,	Kreosote,	Silicea,
Acal. indica,	Drosera,	Lobelia,	Stannum,
Belladonna,	Ferrum,	Lycopodium	Sanguinaria,
Bryonia,	Hepar sulph.,	Lachesis,	Sepia,
Bromine,	Hamamelis,	Mercurius,	Sulphur.
Calc. carb.,	Hypophosphite of Lime,	Nitric acid,	

Dr. Epps, in his work on "Consumption," gives thirty seven remedies, viz:

Aconite,	Causticum,	Ignatia,	Phosphorus,
Arnica,	Cantharis,	Kali carb.,	Pulsatilla,
Arsenicum,	Clematis,	Lycopodium,	Quinine,
Asafoetida,	Cinnamon,	Lachesis,	Rhus tox.,
Belladonna,	Cod liver oil,	Ledum,	Sulphur,
Bryonia,	Graphites,	Merc. sol.,	Spongia,
Baryta carb.,	Hepar sulph.,	Nux vomica,	Sepia,
Calc. carb.,	Helleborus,	Nitric acid,	Veratrum alb.
China,	Ipecac,	Opium,	

Dr. Hugh Hastings, in his "Consumption, it's prevention and cure," gives nineteen remedies, viz:

Aconite,	Bryonia,	Carbo veg.,	Lycopodium,
Amm. carb.,	Calc. carb.,	Digitalis,	Nitric acid,
Arnica,	Causticum,	Dulcamara,	Phosphorus,
Arsenicum,	China,	Ferrum,	Sulphur.
Belladonna,	Cod liver oil,	Kali carb.,	

Dr. E. H. Ruddock, in his work on "Consumption," gives twenty eight remedies, viz:

Aconite,	Calc. phos.,	Iodine,	Nux vomica,
Arsenicum,	Cod liver oil,	Kreosote,	Phosphorus,

Arsenate of	Drosera,	Kali bi.,	Phos. acid,
Soda,	Ferrum,	Laurocerasus,	Podophyllum,
Belladonna,	Hepar sulph.,	Lycopodium,	Pulsatilla.
Bryonia,	Hyoscyamus,	Merc. sol.,	
Calc. carb.,	Ignatia,	Mercurius iod.,	
China,	Ipecac,	Millefolium,	

Dr. Richard Huges, in his "Therapeutics," gives seventeen remedies, viz:

Arsenicum,	Hyoscyamus,	Kreosote,	Phosphorus,
Calc. carb.,	Iodine,	Lycopodium,	Stannum,
China,	Ipecac,	Pulsatilla,	Spongia,
Drosera,	Kali carb.,	Phos. acid,	Sulphur.

Dr. A. Charge, in his "Traitement Homoeopathique, des Maladies des organes de la Respiration," in the section "Phthisic Pulmonaire," gives forty two remedies and fifteen "Medicaments intercurrents," viz:

Amm. carb.,	China,	Lachesis,	Plb. acet.,
Amm. mur.,	Conium,	Lycopodium,	Sanguinaria,
Ars. alb.,	Drosera,	Lysimach.	Sepia,
Ars. iod.,	Eryth. coca,	nummularia	Silicea,
Ars. nat.,	Ferrum,	Merc. sol.,	Silphion,
Bovista,	Hepar sulph.,	Natrium mur.,	Spongia,
Calc. carb.,	Iodium,	Nitric acid,	Stannum,
Calc. phos.,	Kali carb.,	Phellandrium	Sticta,
Calc. sulph.,	Kali iod,	aquaticum,	Sulphur,
Carbo veg.,	Kali nit.,	Phosphorus,	Thuja.
Caustic,	Kreosote,	Plumbum,	

"MÉDICAMENTS INTERCURRENTS"

Aconite,	Belladonna,	Hyoscymus,	Pulsatilla,
Actaea rac.,	Bryonia,	Lactucarium,	Sambucus,

Allium cepa, Digitalis, Laurocerasus, Tartar emetic.
Allium sat., Hydr. ac., Myrtus communis,

Dr. J. Kafka, in his work on "Therapeutics" gives fifty four remedies for tuberculosis of the lungs, twelve of which he has great confidence in, the balance has given him but little satisfaction; they are the following :

Calcarea carb., Chinin sulph., Kali carb., Natrium m.,
China, Hepar sulph., Mercury, Silicea,
Cod liver oil, Iodine, Phosphorus, Sulphur.

MINOR REMEDIES

Aconite, Conium, Lachesis, Sepia,
Apis m., Hyoscyamus, Lycopodium, Stramonium,
Arsenicum, Ignatia, Nux vomica, Thuja,
Belladonna, Kali iod., Pulsatilla, Veratrum alb.

INCIDENTAL REMEDIES

Atropine, Colchicum, Morphine, Secale cor.,
Arnica, Carbo veg., Nitric acid, Sambucus,
Amm. carb., Digitalis, Opium, Sabadilla,
Bryonia, Ergotinum, Phos. acid, Tartar emetic,
Cannabis, Ferrum, Rhus tox., The mineral
Chamomilla, Ipecacuanha, Rheum, springs.
Colocynth, Lactucarium, Sulphuric acid,

A careful study of the above remedies used by the homoeopathic school, reveals the fact, that the real curative agents in consumption have for their starting point, or centre of action, the ganglionic nervous system, the cerebro-spinal remedies being only given for incidental symptoms, and not depended upon as the true curative agents by any of our school. This is strong evidence that the great sympathetic, or vegetative nervous system, is the great receptacle for that fearful destroyer, tuberculosis. Now if this disease has for it's grand centre of action and starting point, the ganglionic nervous system, we at once get a true idea of the class of remedies that should be given to arrest it, their grand centre of action must be on the *same tissues.* This gives us a large number of well tried remedies that will really cure this frightful destroyer. Of course, every remedy in the materia medica will be more or less useful for incidental symptoms, but the *grand curative ones* must be those having a *specific action* upon the great *vegetative* nervous system.

Dr. Frost, of Bangor, Maine, published in the sixth volume of the *American Homoeopathic Review,* Page 145, an article entitled "The Sympathetic and Spinal Systems in relation to Psora," wherein he "advocates the ganglionic system as the fundamental form of life, common alike to the lowest and to the highest species, and this vital principle, peculiar to the ganglionic system, is originally constructive and constantly sustaining all the rest. Hence all that is meant by *constitution* must belong to the ganglionic system, which, in immediate relation to the seminal embryo, precedes both spinal and cerebral organization. In those obscure recesses of nature, the minute, individual and collective ganglia of the sympathetic system, lie concealed, the subtle but persistent germs of health and longevity on one hand, and of disease and premature decay on the other. Here, amid the *primary and most secret springs of life,* ready to flow with them into all the vital organization and into the spinal and cerebral systems, and to perpetuate itself in procreation and conception, lurks the latent, miasm, the aqua tophana of scrofula, or of that hereditary psora, which since Hahnemann's time has remained a questio vexata to the physicians."

And again, page 151: "Instead of being limited to an "itch," suppressed in the person of the sufferer himself or in some of his ancestors, psora *may be regarded as an hereditary taint of constitution.* Doubtless, the skin is the primary and preferred form of development in all chronic as well as all acute disease. The relation between the sympathetic ganglia and the spinal cord is still imperfectly understood. Disease in the great sympathetic, occasions tenderness of the spinous processes, which is sometimes mistaken and unavailingly treated for spinal disease. The *ganglionic* system *contains all the hereditary elements of health and disease,* which later may be considered as *latent* till they begin to be transmitted to some of the organizations which this system supplies. It is believed that the germs of the hereditary dyscrasia, latent in the sympathetic ganglia, may be discovered in the form of minute tubercles in the involuntary organs, in the spinal marrow, and in the brain." With these few remarks, we will commence with first.

GENERAL ATONIC CONDITION OF THE BODY

This symptom may exist from infancy up to manhood, and arises from an undeveloped physical organization; the subject inherits a scrofulous constitution; the thorax is ill formed, flattened and inclined to become contracted; respiration is above the normal standard, and greatly accelerated on slight exertion.

The germ of tuberculosis lies dormant in the organic nervous system, and the most trivial event may kindle the spark into a flame that will not end until death claims the victory.

The treatment of this condition is to strive to get a better development of the body, by insisting upon obedience of all the laws of health, advising a proper selection of food, and the use of gymnastics. During the period of development, gymnastics are invaluable, and their effects are sometimes most miraculous, in developing the muscular system. "A systematic course of exercises which shall especially bring into play the muscles of the chest and keep the body erect, will greatly enlarge the capacity of the chest; the lungs may be made to receive a much larger quantity of air; but it is necessary that this course of health giving exercises should be commenced before a hopeless structural disease already exists, and that it be so directed as not to 'give fatigue and exhaustion in the nervous system out of all proportion to the effect upon the muscles.' The general indication says Dr. C.F. Taylor "will be met by employing the muscles in such a manner that while they are made to act with more or less force, no greater demand shall be made upon the nervous system than can be easily and healthfully responded to."

"The first thing to be attended to and never to be lost sight of for a moment, is the circulation of blood. Feebleness of the heart's action, imperfect respiration, poor quality and small quantity of blood, and especially want of affinity between the blood and the tissues, all conspire to produce the livid countenance, cold extremities, and consequent pectoral congestion and oppression so characteristic of pulmonary consumption. It is advised to act almost wholly and very perseveringly on the extremities, by rotations of the feet, hands, arms, and legs, and by flexions and extensions of the same, *but there should never be any attempts to expand the chest*, till after the peripheric circulation has been improved. After a proper distribution of the fluid has been secured and maintained, improved health is sure to follow."

For full and minute directions on how to use these physical movements, the reader is referred to the works treating particularly upon *gymnastic exercises*.

BREATHING TUBES

The use of breathing as a physical exercise for the lungs cannot be urged upon the patient too strongly. It is a good means of developing the muscles of the chest, and nothing is so beneficial as an habitual custom of taking deep and free inspirations.

The use of *breathing tubes* will soon get the patient into the habit of deep and full inspirations.

HEALTH-LIFT

The use of the *health-lift* is, without doubt, the most important remedial agent that has been devised by man for the cure of a general atonic condition of the body. It is the most thorough, the most expeditious, the safest and easiest method of developing the whole muscular system that can be thought of, for it exercises almost all the muscles in the body simultaneously, at a minimum expense of mental effort. The chief recommendation of this means is, that the apparatus is so *simple* that the most fragile woman, if she can but stand up, can use it with perfect safety. From *six weeks* to two months exercise, spending each day, *ten or twelve minutes* in *health-lift exercise*, will give her not only a strong muscular system, but health also.

Consumptives who have been treated by the *health-lift* have uniformly found their health and strength improved daily, cough and expectoration diminished, appetite improved, pulse became slower and stronger, the capacity of the lungs greater, the mobility of the chest frequently doubled, the circumference greatly enlarged, increase of weight, and all the appearance of returning health.

The *health-lift* apparatus consists substantially of a table or platform, upon which the individual stands between two vertical iron rods, attached to a cross bar below the table; from which the cross bar is suspended by a slogger joint, a notched shaft to which any number of fifty pound iron plates may be keyed. Each vertical rod holds, in a suitable socket, an inclined handle, so shaped to the hand as to give the greatest possible friction surface, whilst it's inclination is such as to throw the weight upon the fleshy cushion of the palm maximum, rather than upon the more bony fingers. Standing thus between the vertical rods, directly over the centre of the weight to be lifted, the heels are separated three or four inches, the toes turned well out, the hands adjusted to the handles, and the knees bent to such an angle as that when the trunk and shoulders are perfectly erect with the shoulders slightly thrown back, arms extended to their fullest limit, and chest expanded, the stature shall be from three to four inches below the usual height. In this position, the knees are slowly and gradually straightened, until the body is perfectly erect, when a line describing the centre of gravity would fall from the point of the shoulder through the hip, knee and ankle joint. In this way the greatest possible amount of muscular tissue is brought into use in it's natural and symmetrical relation; no one muscle, or set of muscles, is unduly exerted, nor are any muscles relaxed. It will be seen that in this way the spinal column is kept perfectly straight, there being no lateral twist or contortion, as in lifting with a cross bar between the legs, which is the usual mode practiced in the gymnasium.

RULES FOR THE USE OF THE HEALTH-LIFT

I—Exercise should be taken usually in the forenoon, about three hours after breakfast—The reason for this involves the physiological law that exercise of function increases the supply of blood in the organs or tissues which is acting—perfect functional activity is impossible, indeed, without a free supply of blood, and, as during this exercise, the muscles "suck up blood like so many sponges," drawing it away from brain, stomach, liver, and every other organ, it is clear, digestion would be interfered with by lifting too soon after eating.

II—Lift slowly—This rule is formed on the fact that the muscles do not contract simultaneously, but some are much more prompt than others—depending upon the amount of use; and as the object is to get the greatest possible bulk

GENERAL ATONIC CONDITION OF THE BODY

of muscular tissue into contraction, it is obvious that this can only be done by giving the more slowly acting muscles time to come into play. This also prevents any undue expenditure of nerve force, economy of which, results in an increase of general vitality.

III—Lift regularly, and as nearly, at the same time each day as practicable—By lifting as nearly as possible at the same hour each day—or every other day—the system reaps the benefit of that compliance with habit which is of so much importance in the economy, and which obtains so largely in our daily life—getting hungry, or sleepy, or waking at given hours, with an almost sentient regularity, and on which the hours of meals and sleep, etc., in health, are based. Hence it is of first importance that this stimulus to the tissue changes, which only lasts a certain time, growing less with varying regularity until it's effect is entirely lost, be renewed at regular periods.

IV—Avoid competition, and do not strive to see how much you can lift.

USUAL EFFECTS PRODUCED BY THE HEALTH-LIFT

Following the exercise most commonly, is a tingling glow over the whole surface of the body, with a sense of buoyancy and vigor which prompts one to want to do something— the exercise seems to have been entirely insufficient—there is a temptation to strike out from the shoulder, to seize the heavy dumb bells, or "skin the cat" on the suspended rings. Instead of spending this increased vitality, however, you are cautioned against doing any of these things: you take it away with you to put it into your daily life and work: the pulse has fallen from five to eight beats per minute, you breath more deeply and fully, the headache is gone, if the feet were cold before, they are now warm. As the exercise is continued, the weak spots develop themselves; the results of former illness or injuries remind you of their existence; probably you find it impossible to raise the weight of yesterday, or even of a week or more previous, you have action where before was stagnation, you may have to go back in your weight, 50, 100, or even 200 lbs, whatever may be the limit of what is now your weakest spot, which is the measure of your strength. Gradually increasing again from this, usually at the rate of ten pounds a day, as you did at first, you reach your old limit and pass it with ease, and have demonstrated that you are a healthier man by so much as you have eliminated that element of weakness.

Sometimes it is attended by pain or discomfort; the more thoroughly circulated blood—in itself healthier and more highly stimulating—arouses sensation a in nerve tissue, hither to dormant.

Each one must be a law unto himself in this matter of weight; some men, and many women lift with benefit only every other day, or lift light and heavy weights on alternate days, and some absolutely need to lift heavy every day. Temperament, occupation, inherent vitality, etc., etc., all must be taken into consideration. No rule can be laid down for any given case, even by the most experienced. Fifty to eighty pounds will frequently tax the strength of the patient at first, but in the course of three or six weeks, three or four hundred pounds can be lifted with ease.

From *ten to twelve minutes of health-lift exercise once a day*, it has been found, after years of experience, to be all that should be taken to get the full benefit of the exercise.

For this atonic condition of the body, change of climate will often be of much value, especially if the patient will

GENERAL ATONIC CONDITION OF THE BODY

go to a place where the atmosphere is very much rarified, such as found in Colorado, New Mexico, and the mountainous portion of North Carolina and Virginia.

Bathing—Frequent bathing, followed by a brisk friction with the flesh brush, will be of much service. Cod liver oil once a day will also be of great value at this early stage of the disease, if persevered in for a long time, especially if the patient is under the influence of such remedies as Calcarea carb., Lycopodium, Phosphorus, Iodium, Silicea and Sulphur.

EMACIATION AND DEBILITY

These two symptoms are so closely united to each other that their treatment will be given together.

The most useful remedies for this condition are Calc. carb., Arsenicum, Iodium, Iodide of Potash, Phosphorus, Silicea, China, Ferrum, Stannum, Sulphur, Kali carb., Lycopodium, Zinc, Cod liver oil, the Health-lift, and a nutritious diet.

> CALCAREA CARBONICA—Leucophlegmatic temperaments, prone to affections of the mucous membranes; dry flabby skin, and in children large, open fontanelles, with large drops of perspiration on the head during sleep. Pale and fair children, with soft flabby muscles, hair dry, looking like tow. Exceedingly sensitive to the least cold air, which seems to go through and through him. Feet cold and damp continually, as if he had cold, damp stockings on.
>
> Walking produces great fatigue, especially walking up stairs; is all out of breath and has to sit down. In women, the menses are too soon, too profuse, and last too long, vertigo on going up stairs. Pains are aggravated by the slightest touch, as from a current of air, noise, excitement, etc.

No remedy in the materia medica acts more profoundly upon the ganglionic vegetative nervous system than Calc. carb., and none is more useful in this destructive disease. In cases of emaciation and debility, where the secondary assimilation of the digested food to blood and tissue does not proceed as it should, we have obstructions "intumescence in the lymphatic and glan-

EMACIATION AND DEBILITY

dular systems, dyscrasial affections of membranous structres, of all the white structres which have but little vitality or blood, and are nourished chiefly by lymph." Development is also imperfect or arrested in the tendons, cartilages, bones and serous membranes.

Emaciation and debility, are the most marked symptoms of Calc. carb., and will always be found one of the most marked symptoms, when this remedy is indicated. Also another marked symptom, if the patient is a child, it has *profuse perspiration* on the head during sleep. Phosphate of lime, in many cases will be the best form to use.

ARSENICUM ALBUM—Rapid and great prostration, with sinking of the vital forces. Extreme emaciation, with great debility, great restlessness, anguish and fear of death. Very weak and prostrated, has a clear countenance, frail look, with a great desire for acids. White, waxy, pale face, with great debility, craves cold water, but the stomach cannot assimilate it; drinks often, but little at a time. Diarrhea of a cadaverous smell, with great enervation after stool. General emaciation with great debility, particularly after midnight.

This remedy is adapted to lymphatic, nervous temperaments, the patient being very sad and irritable. Through the ganglionic system, expecially the solar plexus, it acts particularly upon the alimentary canal. "The organic functions of the whole sympathetic nervous system are stricken down and destroyed from the inmost recesses of vitality. The blood making power of the ganglionic nervous system is completely annihilated by the action of Arsenicum. The poison acts directly on the red corpuscles, diminishing their power of taking up the oxygen supplied to them in the lungs; and the carbonaceous compounds thus unconsumed, deposit themselves in the form of fat. If this direct action on the corpuscles be granted, many of the phenomena of arsenical poisoning become explicable. No wonder the blood is black and non-coagulable, resembling that of malignant fever and cholera. Petechial effusions frequently occur, and the chronic poisoning takes the form of the profound stages of consumption, when we have cold, clammy sweats, great emaciation and debility accompanied with more or less dyspnea, general emaciation, and anasarca.

This remedy will often be called for in the second and last cachexia."

> **IODIUM**—Remarkable and unaccountable weakness with loss of breath when going up stairs. Cachectic, scrofulous people, especially women, with dwindling away of the mammae; they hang down heavily and lose their fatness. Dark brown colour of the face, excessive debility during the menses. Greatly aggravated by motion.

This is one of our most important remedies in confirmed phthisis. It's main action through the ganglionic system is spent upon the lymphatic glandular system.

Dr. Hughes says : "It's true action is one of a depressant character, exerted upon the lacteal vessels and mesenteric glands, giving a sluggish taking up of the fatty elements of the food by the lacteals, and an insufficient elaboration of their contents by the mesenteric glands, and we have at once the most important channel of nutrition choked up and rendered useless. The fatty aliments being those taken up by the lacteals, the emaciation becomes more rapidly apparent than if it had been the albuminous constituents of the diet whose supply was cut off. The action on the glands of which the emaciation of Iodine is thus a prominent instance, displays itself also in the salivary glands, liver, glands of the generative system, and the thyroid. Upon the glands of the generative system it exerts a depressing and atonizing influence. The mammae and testes have more than once wasted away and disappeared under it's use; and a diminution of the functional energy of the ovaries makes it probable that those are similarly affected."

The most marked effects of Iodine are: "Over excitement of the whole nervous system; ebullition of blood and pulsations over the whole body, increased by every effort; trembling, tottering gait; great debility, atrophy; extreme emaciation; general oedema; pulse accelerated, hard and small; hectic fever; variable appetite, either excessive or absent; digestion is very feeble; dyspepsia; suffocation; out of breath on going up stairs, with violent palpitations and cramp like pains about the heart on the least effort." Symptoms are greatly aggravated by motion.

> **KALIUM IODATUM**—This remedy is so closely related to Iodine, that we will not in this place give separate indications, but simply state where we find the symptoms strongly pointing towards it; the patient is saturated with mercury, has had syphilis, and rheumatic symptoms, with much derangement of the mucous membranes. Here we would rather give the Iodide of Potassium the preference.

> **PHOSHORUS**—People with meagre, slender form, fair complexion and strong sexual feelings. Sensation of weakness in the abdomen, that aggravates all the other symptoms. Stools are long, narrow, hard and very difficult to void, or profuse, watery, exhaustive diarrhea pouring away as from a hydrant. Profuse haemorrhages, anaemia, with profuse perspiration and great emaciation.

When the disease is deep seated with much emaciation, great nervous prostration, and more or less complicated with gastric and intestinal disease, Phosphorus will be found of much value. There is much anaemia and deliquescence of the blood, with frequent haemorrhages of dark, fluid blood. The emaciation is accompanied with a dry, hard cough; the expectoration is frequently mixed with blood; the lungs more or less hepatized and much sanguineous infiltration of the parenchyma. There is a great tendency to a watery, exhaustive diarrhea, or much gastric irritability; the tongue is red at the tip and sides; nausea and more or less vomiting.

> **SILICEA TERRA**—Emaciation accompanied with more or less suppuration going on in the lungs. Profuse night sweats. Much perspiration about the head and chest, especially in little children. Terribly offensive sweat on the feet. Hungry, but cannot get down food, it is so nauseous. Great constipation, the rectum has no power to expel the stools, the stool recedes after being partly voided. Great want of vitality, always cold, takes cold at every change of the weather. Greatly constipated before menstruation.

In emaciation and debility where organic changes are taking place, especially suppuration; it has an extraordinary control over the suppurative process, seeming to mature abcesses when desired, and certainly reducing the excessive suppuration to moderate limits.

This remedy is especially adapted to children who are inclined to rachitis, with large bellies and weak ankles; great difficulty in learning to walk. Emaciation, with ulceration of the lymphatic glandular system. The emaciation that calls for Silicea has been brought on by a *long lasting* organic disease of lungs, or some other organ undergoing suppuration.

> **CHINA**—In emaciation where the system has been debilitated by the loss of vital fluids, especially blood, semen, over lactation, leucorrhea, diarrhea, or profuse night sweats. Great distention of the abdomen, not relieved by eructation or dejections. Debilitating diarrhea of undigested food. Emaciation, where debility is the most prominent symptom, from loss of blood. Anaemic people with frequent, exhaustive haemorrhages, long lasting, congestive headaches. Excessive sensitiveness of the skin, with much irritability and sadness. The least draft of air causes great suffering.

EMACIATION AND DEBILITY

In emaciation and debility due to profuse haemorrhages from the lungs, or excessive suppuration, accompanied with night sweats, China will be found of great value.

The cases that especially call for China have many gastric symptoms, one of the most prominent of which is immense distention of the abdomen, it seems to be fully packed with gas, not relieved by eructation or dejection, with much acidity in the stomach. Anaemia with excessive debility from loss of vital fluids. Most of the symptoms of China are aggravated in the evening and at night. It's great action is to cause *debility* of the *trophic* nervous system. Debility is to the nervous system what anaemia is to the blood, and this is the great field for the action of China, or it's alkaloid, the Sulphate of Quinine. It's medicianal effect is to build up and prevent the destruction of nerve tissue. In emaciation and debility from the loss of vital fluids there is great disintegration of nervous tissue; in such states China, and especially the Sulphate of Quinine, contributes wonderfully to the reparative process, in fact, may be called the great *conservator* and builder of the cerebro-spinal nervous system.

> **FERRUM METALLICUM**—Anaemia, with a pale face, emaciation and great debility. Weak persons, the least exertion or motion produces a red, flushed face. Bellows sound of the heart, with anaemic murmurs in the arteries and veins, muscles feeble, and easily exhausted from slight exertion. Lienteria, the food is undigested and painless.

Iron especially affects the blood plasma, decreasing the albumen and red corpuscles, increasing the water in the serum sanguinis, producing anaemia and chlorosis. Diarrhea with stools of mucus and undigested food; the stools are painless, excoriating and exhaustive. Menses intermit two or three days, and then return again; blood pale and watery. General haemorrhagic tendency. Emaciation, with oedematous swelling of the body; cool skin, constant chilliness and evening fever. Symptoms aggravated towards and in the morning, while at rest, especially when sitting still. Amelioration from slow exercise. Emaciation and debility brought on by the abuse of quinine, and alcoholic drinks where there is marked enlargement of the spleen, and anaemia.

> **STANNUM METALLICUM**—Great weakness of the chest, the least exertion puts him all out of breath, can not answer questions, debility centers in the chest; reading aloud, coughing, or the effort to expectorate produces great weakness in the lungs. Feels so weak, can hardly sit down, must drop down suddenly, but can get up very well. Great weakness of the legs, they cannot support the body.

The cases that will be cured by this remedy, will have great prostration of the whole cerebro-spinal nervous system, the most of which seems to centre in the chest.

With the emaciation and debility the patient is apt to have a cough, with profuse, greenish expectoration. Goes up stairs easily, but becomes very faint on coming down. "The pains commence lightly, increase gradually to a vary high degree, decrease again as slowly."—*Hahnemann.*

Debilitating night sweats, in the morning, particularly affecting the neck and chest.

All the symptoms are relieved by walking (except the debility) but return at once during rest.

> **SULPHUR**—Sensation of constant heat on top of the head. Feels very weak and faint from 11 to 12 A.M., she must have her dinner. Early morning diarrhea, driving the patient out of bed, has hardly time to keep from soiling herself. Excoriating discharge from the bowels or urinary organs, especially in children. Feeling of suffocation; must have the doors and windows open. Sudden flashes of heat, which soon pass off with moisture and debility. Great heat in the palms and especially in the soles, wishes to find a cool place for them or puts them out of bed.

Long lingering cases that seem to get almost well, when they relapse again and again.

Great emaciation and debility, with much rattling of mucus in the lungs, and the catarrhal symptoms become worse and worse. Chronic constipation, the stools are hard, dark and dry, expelled with great difficulty, frequently accompanied with bleeding piles, or the patient has chronic diarrhea driving him out of bed early in the morning, with many weak, fainting spells through the day. The skin is full of pimples and eruptions, with a great disposition to excoriation. Offensive, corrosive, ichorous leucorrhea. Chronic uterine haemorrhages, that seem to get almost well, and then return again and again. Menses thick, black, and so acrid that it make's the vulva and legs sore. The child has great voracity, watches eagerly for everything it sees.

Emaciation and debility, with hoarseness and roughness in the throat, and much mucus in the chest. Great dyspnea, shortness of breath and oppression of breathing. Asthma at night.

Tearing pains in the outer parts of limbs, in the muscles and joints, commencing above and running downwards.

Symptoms worse in the evenings, or after midnight. It will often rouse the slumbering vitality, if the proper medicines have failed to produce a favorable effect, especially in acute cases.

KALIUM CARBONICUM—The characteristic of this remedy in long diseases is stitching pains, and the symptoms are all worse in the morning, at 2 or 3 A. M., when at rest, and better in the open air. Great liability to take cold at every change in the weather. Swelling over the upper eyelids in the morning, looking like little sacks.

In emaciation and debility where there is a dry cough, invariably aggravated about 3 A.M., hectic fever and night sweats, with many stitching, darting, shooting, cutting pains, this remedy is invaluable. It seems to act on the system so as to produce dryness of the serous membranes, which gives rise to the stitching pains, the great leading characteristic of the remedy.

Suppuration of lungs, with great emaciation and debility, accompanied by profuse night sweats, affecting more especially, the head and chest.

Excessive dryness of the scalp, with falling off of hair.

Great liability to take cold at every change of the weather. Very irritable, with much anxiety, fear and tendency to start from the least noise. Rheumatic subjects.

LYCOPODIUM CLAVATUM—Great quantities of red sand in the urine. Much pain in the back before urinating, relieved as soon as the urine begins to flow. Constant sense of satiety. Great accumulation of flatus in the stomach and abdomen, much fermentation with sour vomiting. Chronic constipation, stools passed with great difficulty. Loose rattling cough with much emaciation and debility. Constantly taking cold at every change of the weather.

In emaciation and debility, where Lycopodium is indicated there will be many dyspeptic symptoms with an immense accumulation of gas in the stomach and bowels, the stomach is often acrid, and the least quantity of food will seem to fill the patient up to the throat. Great emaciation of the upper part of the body, while the lower portion is enormously distended.

Cough day and night, with expectoration of large quantities of muco-purulent matter.

EMACIATION AND DEBILITY

Night sweats, perspiration cold, clammy, sour, fetid, bloody and sometimes smelling like onions.

The patient is very low spirited, and melancholic; grieves constantly and is excessively irritable.

Dr. Pope thinks there are but few medicines so valuable in consumption as this, when persistently used. The cough, gastric irritation, emaciation and debility are wonderfully mitigated by it.

The symptoms are aggravated at 4 P.M., and at night, or at 9 in the morning.

ZINCUM METALLICUM—Cerebral exhaustion with mental and physical depression, from anaemia of the brain. Incessant and constant fidgety feeling of the feet; must move them constantly.

In emaciation and debility, where there is great debility of the cerebro-spinal nervous system, his remedy is often of great value; it seems to be to the animal nervous system, what Iron is to the blood. Many gastric symptoms, with distended abdomen, and dry, hard, small stools.

Strong sexual desires. Marked weakness and trembling of hands. Profuse perspiration all through night, with an inclination to uncover one's self.

Most of the symptoms are aggravated after dinner.

I now use the hypophosphorous zincum, with better results than in the metallic form.

OLEUM JECORIS ASELLI—Cod liver oil. This is obtained from the liver of the common cod; the process is thus described by Dr. Garrod: "The livers are collected daily, so that there is no trace of decomposition; it is then carefully examined, so as to remove all traces of blood and impurity, and to separate any inferior livers. They are then sliced and exposed to a temperature not exceeding 180° F., till all the oil is drained from them. This is filtered, and later exposed to a temperature of about 50° F., in order to congeal the bulk of the margarine. It is then again filtered, and put into bottles, well secured from the action of air."

Cod liver oil, being the only agent in which the old school has any confidence as a curative agent in tuberculosis, let us first see what the oil really contains.

Dr. Jongh, found the principal constituents of these oils to be *oleate* and *margarate* of *glycerine* possessing the usual properties, constituents of bile such as *fellenic, cholic* and *bilifellinic acids,* and *bilifulvin,* a *peculiar substance* soluble in alcohol, a *peculiar substance* soluble in water, alcohol, or ether; *iodine, chlorine,* and traces of *bromine; phosphoric,* and *sulphuric acids; phosphorus; lime; magnesia, soda, and iron.*

These were found in all the varieties, though not in equal proportions in all, yet it is quite uncertain whether the difference had any relation to their degree of efficacy.

This analysis gives us a compound of twenty different remedies, all of which, it will be seen, act especially upon the *great sympathetic or vegetable nervous* system, the *grand centre* for the action of the *tubercular poison,* and, it in one of the principal remedies used by our school for the cure of tubercular consumption. This analysis also gives us an explanation how cod liver oil cures consumption. First it holds in solution a fine attenuation of lime, iodine, phosphorus, bromine, and a large number of other valuable remedies, and it is nonsensical to think they do not act medicinally.

Our preparations of the same remedies in which we all have such unbounded confidence, contain far less medicine of each one of the ingredients, at the 30th and 200th attenuation, than the oil. We would like to see the chemist who could give the amount of iodine, the 30th or 200th centesimal attenuation contain to the grain or ounce. We are certain that they do act medicinally in those attenuations. A chemist can tell us the quantity of iodine contained in an ounce of oil, but he cannot in an ounce of the 200th attenuation of iodine. Consequently, we must conclude from this, that the beneficial influence exerted by cod liver oil in phthisis, is to a large extent *medicinal.* Secondly, it is also a hightly nutritious and easily assimilable food. In all ages oleaginous substances have been esteemed highly as curative agents in consumption, whether their action was to be attributed to their medicinal, or to their nutritious properties. We now see that it supplies nutriment in a concentrated form, and at the same time holds in solution medicines that are homoeopathic to the tubercular diathesis.

Dr. C.J.B. Williams, in his late work on pulmonary consumption says: "After a quarter of a century's experience, it is the only agent in any degree deserving the title of a remedy in this disease. It's mode of action is still a matter of uncertainty, but we can at least offer some reasonable conjectures. That it is in itself a nutriment cannot be doubted, and that it's nutritious properties go farther than to augment the fat in the body is proved by the well ascertained fact that the muscles and strength also increase under it's use. In fact, it has been proved to increase the proteinaceous constituents of the blood except the fibrin which is diminished; in truth, the beneficial operation of cod liver oil extends to every function and structure of the body. In cases most suitable for it's use, there is a progressive improvement in digestion, appetite, strength and complexion; and various morbid conditions are perceptibly diminished. Thus purulent discharges are lessened, ulcers assume a healthier aspect, colliquative diarrhea and sweats cease; the natural secretions become more copious and the pulse less frequent. It is difficult to comprehend how it can produce such marvellous, manifold salutary effects." (It produces these marvellous effects through the vegetative nervous system). "When we remember that in a teaspoonful of oil we are administering a dose of Iodine equal to a drop and a half of it's 3rd decimal dilution, and that we are generally giving it in cases to which the drug is thoroughly homoeopathic, can we doubt that it exerts a curative action; if we disbelieve this, we have no reason for believing in the action of infinitesimals anywhere. Moreover were it the oleaginous matter *per se* which cures, why should all attempts to find a substitute for the oil of fishes be so unsuccessful?"

In cases that are benefited by the use of Cod liver oil, the nutrition of the body is at fault, and we find the loss of flesh, or emaciation a prominent symptom, with marked debility, or we may have enlargement of the lymphatic glandular system, and swelling of the cervical, or sub-maxillary in little children.

There are three varieties of oil in use; the dark brown, a brown and a pure, pale oil. The latter is the only kind that ought to be used for medicinal purposes. The strong smelling and dark coloured oils owe their offensive properties to the partial decomposition and putrefaction that has taken place before the oil is taken from the livers. Speaking about the various kinds of oil, Dr. Williams says in his work on consumption: "It was not until the pure, pale oil was brought under my notice that the difficulties in administering it gave way; and during the last twenty five years, I have prescribed it (pale oil) for between twenty and thirty thousand patients, and with such success that it was taken without material difficulty by about 95 per cent of the whole number, and of those who took it (90 per cent) derived more or less benefit from it's use. This experience, which is in accordance with that of many of my professional friends, is at least quite as strong as any, that can be adduced in favor of the brown or impure kind of oil, and it does seem absurd to recommend the exhibition of the remedy in it's offensive form, when the pure, fresh oil has been proved to be at least equally efficacious."

To get the full benefit of the oil, it's use must be persevered in for at least several months, and some patients will find it their staff of life, and will have to continue it for their whole lifetime.

To preserve the oil, the bottle should be well corked and kept in a cool place; the oil should not be exposed to the air any longer than it is necessary to take it.

Dr. Mayhofer says: "Cod liver oil justly merits the high reputation which it has acquired in correcting those deficiencies of nutrition commonly comprehended in the terms of scrofulosis and tuberculosis. In patients exhibiting a strumous diathesis, of a slender and lean figure and thin, transparent skin, we generally find combined a frequent weak pulse, great excitability of the nervous system, with high specific gravity of the urine—all signs of an accelerated metamorphosis. It is in this condition that the action of Cod liver oil has obtained it's anti-scrofulous fame. In a short time after its use the angular forms acquire more roundness, and the general susceptibility, as well as the morbid phenomena, gives way to its influence. Scrofulous individuals however, who exhibit a fatty, puffy, leuco-phlegmatic body, swollen nose and upper lip, slowness of the cardiac contractions, defective irritability of the nervous system, and low specific gravity of the urine, far from being benefited by Cod liver oil are the very victims who have been made to swallow it my quarts, and to no purpose. The reason of this is obvious: fat requires nearly double the amount of oxygen for it's combustion (100 : 292.14) to that demanded by albumen (100 : 153.31) and as it evinces a greater tendency for the generation of acid than the latter, acts, when introduced into the organism, the part of a moderator to the metamorphosis of nitrogenous substances. On the other hand, that part of the oleagenous matter which has not furnished it's share towards the production of animal heat by combustion, does so by it's accumulation under the cutaneous surface, or enters as a necessary element into the formation of cells. It is thus evident that Cod liver oil can only be of service when the destructive nutritive process prevails over the constructive one, and that otherwise it's agency must rather increase than diminish a lymphatic tendency of the constitution.

But the virtues of this animal product are, by a great number of physicians, attributed to the measure of Iodine contained in it. There can be no doubt as to the salutary influence exercised by this metalloid over some special scrofulous affections; but this does not destroy the fact that Cod liver oil, like any other fatty substance (the fat of dogs is a popular remedy in Germany for scrofula and phthisis), produces it's best effects on lean persons, who as physiology teaches, consume more oxygen and excretes more carbonic acid and bile than fat ones, while on those who show a disposition to the formation of adipose tissue, it effects a contrary result to that which is desired, in spite of the Iodine which it contains. Cod liver oil is a specific only in a limited number of morbid conditions; in the majority of instances it derives it's importance from it's value as a nutritive agent arresting a preternatural waste."

Dr. Walshe, an allopathic physician, whose authority on this subject, no physician can out rank in any school, draws the following conclusions.

(1) That Cod liver oil more rapidly and more effectually induces improvement in the general and local symptoms than any other known substance.

(2) That it's power of curing disease is undetermined.

(3) That the mean amount of permanency of the good effects of the oil is undetermined.

(4) That it relatively produces more marked effects in the third, than in the previous stages.

(5) That it increases weight in favorable cases with singular speed, and out of all proportion to the actual quantity taken; that hence it must in some unknown way save waste, and render food more readily assimilable.

(6) That it sometimes fails to increase weight.

(7) That in a great majority of cases where it fails to increase weight, it does little good in other ways.

(8) That it does not relieve dyspnea out of proportion with other symptoms.

(9) That the effects traceable to the oil in the most favorable cases are : increase of weight, suspension of colliquative sweats, improved appetites, diminished cough and expectoration, cessation of sickness with cough, and gradual disappearance of physical signs.

(10) That in some cases it cannot be taken either, because it disagrees with the stomach, impairing the appetite (without being itself absolutely nourishing) and causing nausea; or because it produces diarrhea.

(11) That in the former case it may be made palatable by associating with a mineral acid; and in the latter prevented from affecting the bowels by a combination with astringents.

(12) That intrathoracic inflammations and haemoptysis are

contraindications to it's use, but only temporarily so.

(13) Diarrhea if depending on chronic peritonitis, or secretive change, or small ulceration in the ilium is no contraindication to the use of the oil; even profuse diarrhea caused by extensive ulceration of the large bowel, is not made worse by it.

(14) That the beneficial operation of the oil diminishes, *caeteris paribus* directly as the age of those using it increases.

(15) That the effects of the oil are more strikingly beneficial when only a small extent of the lung is implicated in an advanced stage, than where a relatively large area is diseased in an incipient stage.

(16) That where chronic pleurisy, or chronic pneumonia exists on a large scale, the oil often fails to relieve the pectoral symptoms.

(17) That it often disagrees, when the liver is enlarged and probably fatty.

(18) That weight may be increased by it, the cough and expectoration diminish, night sweat ceases, the strength which has been failing remains stationary under the use of the oil, and yet the local disease may all the while be advancing. "Singular proof," says Dr. Walshe, "of the nutritive power of the agent," and, we may add, of it's inefficiency as a medicine.

"This admirable exhaustive summary of the knowledge which is possessed of the subject to which it relates, confirmed, as it has been, by the conclusions of competent observers, shows a wide difference between the anticipations which were indulged respecting the virtues of Cod liver oil and the sober realities of experience. But enough remains to prove that among the remedies that have been proposed for pulmonary consumption, none can be compared with this in efficacy.

More than any other, it mitigates the symptoms of the disease, and delays it's march; while in some cases it appears permanently to arrest the degeneration of tubercles already deposited, and so to improve the nutrition as to prevent the formation of new ones."

—STILLE.

Dr. H.C. Wood says: "There can be no doubt that consumption often commences with catarrh, and is often developed slowly, as the result of frequently "catching cold." Whenever a patient is feeble, pale, somewhat anaemic, complains of his liability to catch cold on the slightest exposure, even though no local disease exists anywhere, or rather because no local disease exists anywhere, there is cause for alarm; and it is of the most vital importance that the patient be put upon a tonic treatment whose basis is Cod liver oil."

Caution—Cod liver oil "should not be administered indiscriminately during the persistence of acute febrile symptoms, congestion, haemorrhages, or any active form of disease; digestion being then impaired, and the mucous membrane irritable, the oil is only likely to increase the disorder. The sphere of Cod liver oil is to remove *exhaustion* and impart general tone; this is best accomplished when active morbid processes and local irritation have subsided, for then the system is in a condition to appropriate a larger amount of nourishment."

—DR. RUDDOCK.

EXHIBITION

Many people and even children have no trouble in taking Cod liver oil, in fact Cod liver oil is taken better by children than by grown people; but, with some the sweetest oil is taken with great difficulty; those who are so sensitive, should take it in the form of *capsules*, or by *inunction*.

One of the best methods I have ever found to administer it is for the patient to suck the juice of a lemon, or chew a little of the lemon skin before taking the oil, and the same after, the taste of the oil is generally all gone in a minute after.

Another good way is to take it floating on a weak solution of *phosphoric acid,* or an infusion of *orange peel,* the quantity of the vehicle should not exceed a tablespoonful, with a teaspoonful of the oil, which should be gradually increased to a tablespoonful for adults, and half the quantity for children.

The oil should be taken morning and night, directly after eating. Experience has taught us that if taken directly after eating it is not so apt to disagree, and rises much less, leaving the appetite free for the next meal. If taken on an empty stomach it leaves for hours a rancid, unpleasant taste, with frequent eructations, tasting of the oil.

Children generally take it very readily; if they should not like it, the best way is to form an emulsion with the yolk of an egg, or mucilage, and flavor it with some syrup, or if the child is very young, the first three decimal triturations can be given in many cases with excellent results, at the same time it can be used on the child by *inunction.*

Dr. Hempel says : "If the stomach is not able to retain the oil, a minute portion of common salt, taken both before and after the dose of oil, will sometimes enable the stomach to bear this remedy when all other devices fail."

Dr. Ruddock says : "Probably the best method of rendering the oil palatable is to have it made up into bread, as it is then scarcely tasted. The proper proportion is two to four tablespoonfuls of the oil to one pound of dough. Patients to whom we have recommended this method of taking the oil assure us that it is pleasant, digestible, and as efficacious when in this as in any other way.' "Small pieces of ice in each dose of oil also render it almost tasteless."

"It's assimilation is promoted and it's beneficial action greatly enhanced, by the addition of ten drops of the first dilution of *Iodium* to each pint of oil. This addition is especially recommended in phthisis pulmonalis, and atrophy."

"Claret is another vehicle for Cod liver oil. The oil should be poured upon the wine, so that it does not touch the glass, but floats as a large globule; in this way it may be swallowed untasted."

A correspondent of the *Lancet* suggests the following method of taking Cod liver oil. "Take one orange and divide it into two equal parts; squeeze the juice of one half into a cup; pour the oil upon it, then squeeze the juice of the other half very gently on the oil. By swallowing the whole, cautiously, even the least taste of oil is not experienced."

Dr. Buchner, in his essay on "Air and Lungs," adverts to the fact that, in England they burn Cod liver oil in several light houses; and that a number of light house keepers, who had been threatened with phthisis pulmonalis, before entering upon the duty above mentioned, inhaled day after day, the air of the lantern impregnated with the volatile parts of the oil, became fleshy and robust. I have acted on the above hint for the past five or six years. In all my prescriptions of Cod liver oil I have directed the inhalations of the vapors arising from *gently* heated (not burned or scorched), crude Cod liver oil and have in more than one case, seen happy results. I direct over a tin dish, filled with sand, and heat the bottom of this either by a stone, or other convenient means. To some the effect is very soothing and grateful. I remember only one instance in which the inhalation of the fumes was at once very distasteful and nauseating, that of a young lady whose health failed repeatedly whenever she lived in New Bedford (near salt water), and gained on her going west to Illinois." G.F. Matthes. *New England Medical Gazette*, vol. 6, p. 6.

I have tested the fumes of the oil as given above, and am pleased with it's action. Inhaling the fumes all night during sleep, will be found of much value in the first stages of phthisis.

Latest Modification of the Cod Liver Oil Emulsion—We have several times called attention to an emulsion of Cod liver oil and phosphoric acid. The last report of the Utica Insane Asylum contains a formula for an emulsion that has long been in use in that institution, and to which our attention was first called by Dr. Andrews. We have experimented considerably with various modifications of the original prescription. The latest formula, and one that suits us better than any other, is the following :

R_x Cod liver oil......................iv. oz.
    Glyconin......................ix. dr.

Glyconin is made by thoroughly triturating glycerine and the yolk of an egg, in equal parts. Add to the glyconin thirty drops of the essential oil of bitter almonds; then add the oil to the glyconin *very slowly,* drop by drop, stirring vigorously all the time. The success of the emulsion depends on the thoroughness with which this task is performed.

Then add—

Jamaica Rum............................ii. ozs.

(Jamaica rum seems to cover the taste better than sherry wine, which has usually been employed).

Dilute Phosphoric acid..........................oz. ss. to oz. i.

The average dose is one tablespoonful after meals, being regulated mainly by the phosphoric acid.

The above combination is a most excellent brain and nerve food. If properly prepared it does not separate, keeps for a long time, and is rather agreeable to the taste. If need be, pyrophosphate of iron can be added, or strychnine, or Fowler's Solution. We have used it especially in hysteria and allied affections, and in organic diseases of the nervous system it is also valuable. Consumptives frequently take it in preference to Cod liver oil. As Cod liver oil has a somewhat unpalatable name, it is sometimes better, in prescribing for nervous patients, to call this the phosphoric emulsion. The fishy odor cannot be entirely neutralized; but for those who are not familiar with Cod liver oil, neither the odor nor taste of this emulsion, when well made, suggests the presence of the oil.—*Arch. Electrology and Neurology.*

As to the kind of diet the patient should use while taking the oil Dr. Williams says. "With some individuals the oil agrees so well and improves their digestion so much, that they require little or no restriction in diet, but this is not the case with the majority. The richness of the oil does prove more or less a trial, sooner or later, to most persons, and to diminish this trial as much as possible, it obviously becomes proper to omit, or reduce all other rich and greasy articles of diet. All pastry, fat meat, rich stuffing, and the like should be avoided, and great moderation should be observed in the use of butter, cream and very sweet things. Even milk in any quantity is not generally borne well during a course of oil, and many find malt liquor too heavy, increasing the tendency to bilious attacks. A plain nutritious diet of bread, fresh meat, poultry or game, with a fair proportion of vegetables, a little fruit, and a moderate quantity of liquid at the earlier meals, commonly agrees best, and facilitates the exhibition of the oil in doses suffcient to produce it's salutary influence in the system."

KOUMISS OR MILK WINE
Fermenting Milk

This natural dietetic remedy has been used extensively by the inhabitants of Tartary, in *consumption,* and diseases where emaciation is a marked feature, with most marvelous effects; in fact with such success, that scrofula and consumption are almost unknown to them, and travellers from all parts of Europe, suffering with phthisis, go into their country to submit themselves to a course of Koumiss, many of whom have returned in perfect health. The success in phthisis has been so great that the imperial government of Russia has established, and supports institutions devoted to the manufacture of Koumiss, and yet here, in progressive America, Koumiss, with all it's virtues, is nearly unknown to the profession; but few things in nature have eluded the keen eyed American, and why has this? Fermenting milk is the most easily digested food known to the physician, containing all the elements of pure milk, consequently contains about all the elements of the human body, it becomes our responsibility as physicians to thoroughly investigate all it's properties, especially if it is of such value in arresting tuberculosis.

Dr. Jarotzki, gives the following reciepe to make Koumiss (Kumiss) :

"Take one tablespoonful of pure honey or golden syrup; eight ounces of brewer's yeast; four ounces of wheat flour; mix thoroughly and add a cup of fresh, tepid milk; make a dough of it, and put it in a warm place, to remain over night. In the morning wrap it in a clean cloth, and place it in an earthen, or china vessel; add to it eight pints of tepid, fresh milk; cover the vessel with a woollen cloth and put it in a warm place, stir it thoroughly several times during the day with a wooden spoon, and in two or three days the fermentation will take place, and fresh Koumiss is produced. Take out two or three pints for the first day's use, and at the same time add the same quantity of fresh, tepid milk. Stir it thoroughly and let it ferment again. Repeat this process from day to day, until the taste becomes more acidulous and the fermentation ceases, when new yeast has to be made again. Koumiss is therefore a *fermenting*, and not a completely fermented milk."

Since writing the above, I have succeeded in getting from my friend, A. Arend, Esq., of 521 W. Madison street, Chicago, the following method to prepare new Koumiss from the old. Mr. Arend is the only chemist, I believe, in the United States, who has really succeeded in making good Koumiss, and he experimented one year before he considered himself qualified to make a good article of the milk-wine. It is made with such difficulty that it requires the nicest manipulation and the most careful attention to all the minor details to succeed.

"The only mode of preparing good Koumiss is that followed in every Tartar household. The manipulation is the same for both mare's milk and cow's milk Koumiss.

Mix one part of the old Koumiss, with five parts of fresh milk, warmed to a temperature of 70° F.; put into a churn and agitate with a churn stick lively at short intervals for a space of three hours; by this time the fermentation is engendered and the fresh Koumiss is ready for bottling; after bottling put in a cool place for twenty four or forty eight hours, when it is ready for use."

To prepare new Koumiss, he uses Dr. Jarotzki's reciepe, as noted above, with some exceptions.

This, the most assimilable of nutriments, contains 980 grains of solid respiratory and plastic food to the quart.

An analysis by Wanklyn, a London chemist gives the following result from a quart of Koumiss.

"Water	10,662	grains
Alcohol	192	,,
Casein and albumen	128	,,
Lactose	582	,,
Lactic acid	130	,,
Fat	36	,,
Ash	90	,,
Carbonic acid	180	,,
	12,00	

"The ninety grains of ash contains approximately 60 grains of phosphate of lime and 30 grains of mixed chlorides of sodium and potassium.

The physical and chemical characteristics of Koumiss render it an aid upon which the physician can rely with great confidence, for the treatment of extreme debility, and all the phases of impending marasmus."

Koumiss not only contains a large proportion of lactic acid, which is a prime constituent of the gastric juice; but holds the casein in that state of vitality which gives it the property of metamorphosing itself and the other constituents of the milk into healthy lymph and blood.

"The process of double fermentation in the preparation of Koumiss does nearly all the preliminary work of digestion, that otherwise must be performed by the stomach. There is no other derivative of milk, or any other substance, that possesses the same advantages; for, containing all the elements of nutrition, and in just that proportion which is necessary to maintain a healthy life, it may constitute a sole diet in cases of disease."

It's great sphere of usefulness is in *emaciation*, similar to Cod liver oil.

Koumiss gives the best results in the first stages of consumption, with emaciation, shortness of breath, tiredness, loose cough, haemoptysis, night sweats, diarrhea and great debility.

"The original Koumiss of the Tartars is made from mare's milk, but chemical research, and the experience of the last ten years proved that cow's milk is an equally good raw material, if not better, and there is no doubt that cow's milk Koumiss gives highly successful results in proper cases, as shown in the Koumiss cures of Odessa, Warsaw, Cracow, St. Petersburgh, Berlin, Dresden, London, & c."

This sparkling and nourishing beverage should be taken like any other food, when the desire for it is felt, and in sufficient quantities to nourish the body.

"The quantity to be taken at a time should be suited to the individual, age and condition of the partaker; if the stomach be irritable, as is generally the case in debilitated constitutions, but a small quantity, for instance a wine glass full, should be taken at once, and this quantity is frequently repeated, until as much as one half or one quart bottle is consumed in a day. As the patient grows stronger and accustomed to this new diet, he will learn to relish the Koumiss and he will be able to take one half, or one gobletful, or more at a time, and as much as two or three quarts in day."

HOW TO KEEP KOUMISS—It has a sweetish sour taste; when at rest, sometimes it separates in severals layers. It then requires to be shaken before using, in order to mix all particles uniformly. If kept in a cool place, between 40° F. and 50° F., Koumiss will remain good for months.

In a temperature exceeding 60° F. it will soon become unpalatable, and unfit for use. In winter, spring or fall when the temperature of the atmosphere does not exceed 60° F. it may be kept in a cool cellar, protected against frost; in summer, when the temperature is above 60° F., Koumiss must be kept on ice.

HOW TO OPEN A BOTTLE OF KOUMISS—Koumiss being very effervescent, requires careful handling in order to prevent waste or damage to surrounding objects. Shake it up well, then allow it to rest for five minutes, the bottle standing; place a pitcher by the side of the bottle, cut the string, remove the cork quickly, and immediately hold the mouth of the bottle, the bottle itself being slightly inclined upward, over the pitcher, and let the liquid work out by it's own force. When all the force is expended, set the bottle down, take what is needed for immediate use from the pitcher, and pour the balance back into the bottle.

A more convenient way is to draw the Koumiss by means of a champagne tap. By using the tap, waste is obviated, and any desired quantity may be drawn at a time, and the full sparkling liquid is retained to the last drop.

Hoping that this short note of *milk wine* will be the means of causing many to use the nourishing beverage to the great benefit of many suffering invalids, I will refer the reader to larger works devoted wholly to Koumiss. Having seen it's salutary effects in my practice, I am anxious that every physician should give his patients the benefit of this *fermenting milk.*

EXTRACT OF MALT

The extract of malt is a very valuable auxiliary in the treatment of phthisis, bronchitis, scrofula, dyspepsia and general debility. Prof. Niemeyer, and Dr. Aiken recommend it very highly as a nutritious tonic, in fact many physicians use it instead of Cod liver oil.

"A single dose of Trommer's extract contains a larger quantity of the soluble constituents of malt than is found in a pint of the best ale, and as it is prepared without being allowed to ferment, it is absolutely free from alcohol and other products of that process.

"In Germany, extract of malt is extensively employed as a substitute for Cod liver oil in pulmonary consumption. The combined experience of the medical world has nevertheless placed the oil on a basis of unrivalled excellence. Where, however, patients have taken the oil for a long time and become tired of it, or it is no longer well borne, and also in the case of those who cannot take the oil, the malt may be employed as a very efficient remedy.

DOSE—It should be taken three times a day, about one tablespoonful for an adult, and half the quantity for a child.

HÆMOPTYSIS

Pneumorrhagia, or pulmonary haemorrhage, generally is a source of great alarm to the patient; but usually, we might say, in great majority of cases, the haemorrhage is a sanguineous exhalation from the mucous membrane of the lungs, and in itself is not a dangerous symptom, but rather an indication that changes are going on in the lungs that will eventually result in fatal tuberculosis. Passive haemoptysis is more intractable than active haemorrhage. When the haemorrhage comes from the lung tissue itself, the symptoms are more violent, and may prove suddenly fatal.

The principal remedies for haemoptysis and pneumorrhagia are Aconite, Veratrum viride, Hamamelis, Millefolium, Ipecacuanha, Phosphorus, Ferrum, Arnica, China, Belladonna, Pulsatilla, Crocus, Trillium, Sanguinaria and Sulphur.

> **ACONITUM NAPELLUS**—Great restlessness, agitation and fear of death, marked congestion of blood in the lungs, with great anxiety. Symptoms aggravated at night; sleeplessness and constant tossing about; especially if brought on in dry, cold air; short dry, titillating, croupy cough.

Active and sudden cases of haemoptysis or pneumorrhagia, when there is much hyperemia of the lungs, after a violent fit of passion, or severe exertion of the lungs. Animated people, with a plethoric habit of body, bright complexion, and disposition to palpitations of the heart. The blood is expectorated with a hacking, dry cough, which torments the patient continually; burning, stinging pains in the chest, the cheeks are flushed; pulse much excited, with great anguish and restlessness; copious discharge of bright red blood, sometimes without much coughing; the face is pale, with an expression of agony in the countenance. The disturbed condition of the mind, with great mental anguish, is the predominating symptom when Aconite is indicated.

> **VERATRUM VIRIDE**—Intense hyperemia of the lungs, with a hard, full, quick, bounding pulse; short rapid respirations, accompanied by more or less gastric symptoms, sudden haemoptysis.

In sudden cases of haemorrhage from the lungs, where the pneumo gastric nerve is more or less implicated. No remedy has such an absolute control over the circulation, by the use of large enough doses of *Squibb's Fluid Extract,* to produce slight nausea. Active haemorrhages can be controlled at will, but in passive haemorrhages it is useful. In active haemorrhages from the lungs, this remedy only has to be given to be appreciated.

> **HAMAMELIS VIRGINIANA**—Especially called for in nervous, passive haemorrhages, the blood is dark and comes into the mouth without any effort, like a warm current out of the chest. Tickling cough, with a taste of blood on waking.

In haemorrhages from the lungs, or any other organ, no remedy has given the profession at large such unvarying and brilliant cures.

Dr. Hughes thinks "the haemorrhages it cures depend rather upon the state of the blood vessels, than that of the blood." We believe, it cures haemorrhages by it's specific action upon the muscles of the capillary blood vessels, causing them to contract.

When the blood comes from the pulmonary mucous membrane, this is well nigh a specific, but if the haemorrhage is due to a rupture of one or more blood vessels from deep ulceration, Aconite, Veratrum viride or Millefolium will be more appropriate.

MILLEFOLIUM—Haemoptysis in tuberculosis, brought on by violent exertions, either active or passive.

This remedy has a special action upon the vascular capillary circulation, controlling active or passive haemorrhages to a marvellous extent.

Hartmann says: "In almost every variety of haemorrhage, and likewise in pulmonary haemorrhage, Millefolium is a splendid and indispensible remedy. More especially in the case of robust and fleshy persons; the spitting of blood is unattended with cough, or the cough is very slight and is caused by the newly accumulating blood; at the same time there is bubbling up in the chest, with a sensation as if warm blood was ascending in the throat, gradually increasing in intensity until blood is raised."

Spitting of blood, with violent palpitations of the heart and much excitement, accompanied with a feeling of great oppression in the chest, active haemorrhages from deep ulcerations in the lungs.

IPECACUANHA—Haemorrhages from all the orifices of the body, with great and long continued nausea, great weakness and an aversion to food. Haemoptysis from the slightest exertion. Much rattling and bubbling of blood and mucus in the bronchial tubes.

For acute haemorrhages, no remedy is used more frequently than Ipecac., and thousands of patients have been cured by

HÆMOPTYSIS

this remedy alone. The great key for it's selection is *great* and *long continued nausea.*

Spasmodic, suffocative cough; asthmatic breathing; blood very dark, and mixed with mucus.

Much rattling of mucus and blood in the bronchi.

Constant taste of blood in the mouth.

The action of Ipecac. in controlling haemorrhages, closely resembles Digitalis; they both arrest the haemorrhage through their action upon the par vagum. If there is any organic disease of the heart so as to cause obstructions to the circulation, Digitalis and especially it's active principle Digitaline, should be preferred. Digitaline is a remedy of untold value in many pulmonary affections, especially if accompanied with a loose, rattling cough and intermittent pulse. It should be given in the 3d. decimal or centesimal trituration.

> **PHOSPHORUS**—Sensation of weakness and emptiness in the abdomen, it is so distressing that it aggravates all the other symptoms. Stools long, narrow and expelled with great difficulty. Fatty degeneration of the liver, with much jaundice. Strong sexual desire, or impotence from sexual abuse. Tightness across the chest, with dry cough, or rusty spots raised with great difficulty. Hard, teasing, dry cough, with a sensation as if cotton was in the throat. Slight wounds bleed much. Tall, slim, nervous temperaments.

This is one of the most valuable remedies we have in haemorrhages. Dr. W. Arnold, of Heidelberg says: "The changes occasioned by it in the blood, and through the blood in the whole organism, have been over looked for a long time. In numerous cases of poisoning by means of Phosphorus matches, and by Phosphorus paste, the changes in the blood are too conspicuous to remain unnoticed any longer. The facts gained in this way were so often confirmed by numerous and of trepeated experiments upon animals that now they are generally accepted. Almost all observers speaking on this subject, describe the blood as being dark, even black, and of fluid consistency. As a rule it is thin, flowing, more rarely of molasses like, or of a more thick flowing appearance. In a coagulated state it has been observed so rarely and exceptionally, and then only in a few single parts of the body that we are justified in assuming that the coagulation cannot be taken as an effect of the *Phosphorus*, but is dependent upon other conditions. Upon the whole, the blood is more fluid if *Phosphorus* does not kill quickly, but has a chance to effect changes in the blood in consequence of a more lasting action for several days. These changes, however, frequently set in very rapidly, if *Phosphorus* has been taken in the form of a solution, as, for instance, in butter, fatty oils, or ether.

"The results of microscopic investigation of blood offer important disclosures. *Phosphorus* occasions an important change in the blood discs, their decrease in consistency and circumference is very conspicuous. They become smaller, more extensible, and consequently can assume different forms. They change their form in many ways, esecially in their passage through narrow vessels, and in their proportion to each other. One might say, that *Phosphorus* acts as a dissolvent upon the blood discs. This action touches the blood cell membrane more than the nucleus. Greater luster, a less granular appearance, irregular and less distinctly defined outlines, are the most conspicuous changes in the blood discs which can undoubtedly be ascribed to the direct action of *Phosphorus*. That these changes take place on account of immediate action, can be proved in this way : I let *Phosphorus* oil act upon the blood under the microscope, and thus I witnessed changes in the blood discs, slighter in degree, it is true, yet entirely similar to those observed from the application of *Phosphorus* during life. In this way I was able to follow up the successive dissolution of the blood discs. This dissolution was not as great as under the continued action of *Phosphorus* in the living organism, and undoubtedly, for the reason that not so intimate and lasting a contact with the blood took place.

"Besides several other observers, *Rummel* testifies to a change in the blood, perceptible under the microscope. He could not find a single coloured corpuscle, but only colourless discs in the blood of a hen, poisoned by *Phosphorus*, and *Voit* made the same observations on a dog, into whose vena cruralis he had injected *Phosphorus*. According to *Rummel*, the destruction of blood discs is the most essential phenomenon when *Phoshorus* has been introduced into the stomach, as well as when directly mixed with the blood by means of injections. The blood discs separate into haematin and globulin. The former floats as a purple coagulum in the plasma, or may according to the conditions present, even be dissolved therein, while the form of the latter is still preserved. Another observation of *Rummel* is very worthy of notice for the explanation of haemorrhages after *Phosphorus* poisoning. If a rabbit, into whose vena cruralis *Phosphorus oil* had been injected, was held head downwards, he soon saw red coloured plasma, which under the microscope was free from any blood discs, flow from the nose. The blood in this dissolved state had passed through the walls of the vessels. On opening a vessel, numerous well preserved blood discs could still be found.

"To judge from the haemorrhages and ecchymosis, so frequently, and, we may say, almost constantly observed in *Phosphorus* poisoning, and from the often confirmed curative action of small doses of *Phosphorus* in morbus maculosus, and many haemorrhagic changes in the blood, must exist and what are they? This question is partly answered by the observations of *Friedreich*. He noticed in a young man afflicted with haematuria, on whose lower extremities oedema, petechae, in short, an exanthema of an exquisitely haemorrhagic character, had made their appearance, that the blood discs, passing with the urine, were essentially changed. They were normal as to form and size only in small numbers, but frequently, very abundantly formed. Many of them were oblong-oval and presented compressions as from ligatures, and so much so, as even to assume the shape of baker rolls. With others, a division into two uneven halves seemed to be taking place. Quite a few had already separated themselves completely and were divided, and this went on until finally blood discs of the most minute form—molecular blood discs, so to say—were formed. This process of division could not only be understood from the results of microscopic examinations, but also be observed directly. The whole left the impression, as if the blood discs consisted in a semi-solid, almost oil like substance, without any external membrane. Even in a case of sarcoma of the kidneys, *Friedreich* has repeatedly seen the above described division of the red blood discs into molecular forms. The red blood discs of anaemic, hydraemic, leukemic, marasmic and strumous individuals, drawn by *Daman*, completely resemble a number of forms presented by *Friedreich*."

This striking resemblance in the change of blood, especially blood discs, after poisoning with *Phosphorus* shows us why it is of such wonderful efficacy in the cure of haemorrhages.

We once cured a case of haemorrhage from the lungs in a tuberculous subject with *Phosphorus,* when the patient had well-nigh bled to death. Without any effort on the part of the patient the blood would rise into his mouth, so that a quart dish would be filled in half an hour, faintness would come on, and the haemorrhage would cease for twenty four hours, and then suddenly come on again. The man was so weak at the end of two weeks that he could not speak above a whisper. Aconite, Hamamelis, Millefolium, Belladonna and Ipecac. all had been tried faithfully and failed. After commencing the use of Phosphorus he had no more haemorrhage, and made a quick convalescence. He remained well for one year, and then died with pulmonary tuberculosis, without any return of the haemorrhage. This confirms *Raue's* observation, "Profuse haemorrhage, pouring out freely, then ceasing for some time."

It is particularly adapted to tall, slender people, with lively perceptions, and inclined to stoop over forward.

> **FERRUM METALLICUM**—Weakly persons with a fiery red face; the least emotion produces a fiery red face, anaemia with great debility, pale face and lips. Haemoptysis, better when walking slowly. Lienteria, undigested stools, without pain. Chlorosis; watery leucorrhea. Great variability of the mind. Oedema of the feet and legs, with a bloated face, and great debility.

In those cases where the blood plasma is impoverished the albumen and red corpuscles are decreased and water in the serum sanguinis.

Great paleness of the increased membranes, especially that of the mouth.

The least mental emotion produces a red flushed face.

Haemorrhagic tendency, with flying pains in the chest.

"Always better from walking slowly about, not withstanding weakness, obliges the patient to lie down. Quick motion and talking brings on cough, with pain between the shoulders; the face has a yellowish tint; sleep is poor at night, and there is frequent palpitations of the heart."

Bellows-sound of the heart, and anaemic murmur in the arteries and veins.

Especially adapted to cachectic and leucophlegmatic individuals, and to diseases where the vegetative system is involved.

"Oedematous swelling of the body; cool skin; constant chilliness, and evening fever, likening hectic fever."—*Hempel.*

The slightest exertion exhausts the patient.

> **ARNICA MONTANA**—Traumatic hæmoptysis. The patient feels sore as if bruised. The bed on which he lies feels too hard; keeps continually changing from place to place. Face hot, while the body and limbs feel cool. Myalgic pains of the intercostal muscles.

Hæmoptysis in weakly people greatly troubled with many muscular pains; the pains occur in all the voluntary muscles or their tendinous prolongations.

Hæmoptysis in people who are subject to boils, and extravasations of blood into the cellular tissue, especially if from some mechanical cause.

The extravasations are quickly taken up by the venous capillaries.

Eructations of putrid gases, as if from rotten eggs.

Hæmoptysis from slight physical exertions, with a constant tickling cough starting from the sternum.

"Particularly useful in venous, plethoric, not very robust individuals; the respirations are very much opressed during the bleeding; the patient is very much disposed to vomit; the attack is caused from every slight exertion, especially in young people." Hartmann.

The expectoration is generally dark red, and raised without much effort.

HÆMOPTYSIS

CHINA—Patient has lost a large quantity of blood, and is worse every other day. Sensation of great distention in the abdomen, not relieved by eructations or dejections. Sour stomach, with debilitating, watery diarrhea, aggravations at night, copious night sweats.

Hæmoptysis in people who have lost much blood, with singing in the ears, and fainting.

Long lasting, congestive headaches, worse at a certain time every day.

Great anæmia from loss of blood, where debility is the prominent symptom.

BELLADONNA—Hæmoptysis with a dry, teasing, spasmodic cough.

Hæmorrhage comes on suddenly, and is worse in the evenings. In robust, plethoric people, catarrhal hæmoptysis, in plethoric people.

This remedy is "particularly applicable in robust, plethoric individuals, and for congestions towards the head, without any cardiac irregularities being complained of; also more particularly if the hæmorrhage was the result of an incipient catarrh." Baehr.

In tubercular hæmorrhage Baehr has no confidence in Belladonna, but if it is vicarious, or at the critical age, he has great confidence in it's medicianal virtues.

Expectoration of bright red blood, with great congestion of blood to the chest, aggravated by motion, with a throbbing headache.

PULSATILLA PRATENSIS—Much chilliness with expectoration of dark, coagulated blood, vicarious menstruation. Menses suppressed. Inclined to diarrhea. Symptoms aggravated in the evenings. Great craving for fresh air, must have the doors and windows open; feels like suffocating in a warm room.

Patients that are very tearful; weeps at everything, whether joyful or sorrowful. Hæmoptysis, with a loose, rattling cough, the bronchi seem loaded with mucus and blood. Hæmoptysis in women who have suppression of the menses. Sub-acute hæmoptysis with dark, venous blood, especially in females who are constantly chilly.

More especially adapted to females, but acts well on both sexes.

CROCUS SATIVUS—Hæmoptysis where the blood is dark and stringy, with much mental dejection. On raising a clot of blood, long strings droop from it.

Passive hæmoptysis is worse evenings. Acts better in women, subject to uterine hæmorrhage of dark coagulated blood; as it is discharged, it forms into long strings. Great debility and palpitations of the heart.

SULPHUR—Frequent flashes of heat, which pass off with moisture and debility. The top of the head is continually hot. Early morning diarrhea, or obstinate constipation. Stools acrid producing excoriation. Ichorous discharges from the nose, vagina or anus. Chronic hæmoptysis; seems to get almost well, when it returns again and again for weeks. Has many weak, faint spells. Heat in the chest with bloody expectoration. Mental symptoms, everything looks beautiful which the patient takes a fancy to, with happy dreams; constant heat in the soles of the feet, puts them out of bed of find a cool place for them; weak faint spells, cannot wait for dinner.

This remedy will be found of great value in those cases that often seem to get almost well, when relapses occur again and again, day after day for a long time.

The cough is loose and rattling, with a suffocative feeling, wants the doors and windows open, craves fresh air so much.

HÆMOPTYSIS

Often has weak, faint spells around 11 A. M.; cannot wait for dinner.

Bends forward when walking, does not walk erect.

Great disinclination to being bathed.

Diseases caused by suppressed eruptions, especially the itch.

Adapted to lymphatic constitutions, disposed to constipation and hæmorrhoids, or to people with chronic morning diarrhea.

There are many remedies that may be useful in hæmoptysis, such as: Trillium, Erigeron, Gallic acid, Ergot, Ustilago maydis, Senecio aureus, Carbo veg., Terebinth., Conium, Opium, Tartar emetic, Hyoscyamus, Drosera, Nitric acid, Sulphuric acid, Collinsonia, Apocynum, Sanguinaria, Cactus, Rhus tox., Lycopodium, Lycopus, Stannum, Calc. carb., Calc. phos., Sepia, Lachesis, Ledum, Arsenicum, &c., &c.

For the special indications of the above remedies, the reader is refered to the materia medica. Usually, however, one or two of the above mentioned remedies will be all that is required.

PRACTICAL EXPEDIENTS

—Dr. Ruddock says :—"The subcutaneous injection of Morphia will control the hæmorrhage almost instantly in a majority of cases."

The cautious use of cold water, or ice, in severe cases, we believe is of much service. The ice should be put into a bladder so as to keep the patient from getting wet, and there should be a towel folded in several thicknesses and laid upon the chest, the bladder of ice is placed upon the towel, and not on the chest. We have seen great benefit from the use of ice applied in this manner.

Ice may be sucked freely, but the better way is for the patient to swallow small pieces of ice and let it dissolve in the stomach, in close contact with the lungs.

Dry cupping has been found of signal service in profuse hæmoptysis. It's action is immediate and decisive. The cups should be applied over the chest, and in the inter-scapular and scapular region.

STYPTICS—Such as Gallic acid, Acetate of Lead, Tannic acid, Sulphuric acid, Alum, Perchloride of Iron and Ergot of Rye, are the principal styptics depended upon in the old school practice. I have never used them and cannot judge their merits.

The Hydrate of Chloral might be of much value as a palliative. The patient must be kept quiet in bed if possible, and his mind free from all excitement. The room should be cool, and his beverages should also be cool, and free from alcoholic stimulants. The diet should consist of cold beef tea, chicken broth, milk, cold tea, coffee, &c., &c.

DIET—A very important item in the treatment of phthisis is the *diet* of the patient. It should be very nutritious and of a non-stimulating nature.

We believe that stimulating food, such as all kinds of liquors, are instead of a benefit, and actual *injury* to the patient. Stimulating drinks lash the digestive organs into an excited feverish state, when there is fever in the system already free from disease.

A small quantity of nutritious, easily digested food, should be taken at a time, on account of the little gastric juice secreted, from the feverish condition of the system.

"Dr. Beaumont observed that there is always disturbance in the stomach when more food has been received than there is gastric juice to act upon it; *i.e.,* a condition induced similar to that which is present in fever, namely, that the gastric juice is not being able to act on the undigested food, the stomach is irritated just as if the food had been introduced into the stomach when the system was in a febrile state.

"If to these facts to the fact already referred to is, that the gastric juice combines with only a given quantity of aliment, it becomes apparent that in weak stomachs, and in persons laboring under disease, the supply of gastric juice being diminished by the state of disease, the evils of taking a large quantity of food must be indeed great." (Constipation, by J. Epps, M.D.)

The patient cannot be too cautious with his diet. Hunger being dependent upon a state of the brain, it may be so irritated as to cause a false hunger, and whatever is fancied cannot be indulged in, for serious results may follow, especially if the digestive organs are implicated.

MILK is an article of diet we greatly prize in phthisis, and all writers on consumption esteem it highly, especially the milk of *asses*. Goats' milk has also gained considerable reputation.

Many physicians recommend the use of lime water and milk.

We believe the reason that *milk* has given such satisfaction in phthisis is because it is so easily digested. The intestinal canal cannot tolerate solid food, but the milk is assimilated into the tissues with the greatest ease.

Soups made from beef, mutton, veal, oysters, &c., &c., will also be found of great value.

When milk disagrees, the *Koumiss* will frequently be a luxury to the patient (see *Koumiss*).

FISH is another article of diet of great value in this disease, and often ought to be indulged in, for we believe it builds up the nervous tissues, especially the ganglionic nerve globules, which we believe is the starting point of this fatal disease. Fish eaters are "especially strong, healthy and prolific. In no other class than that of fishers do we see larger families, handsomer women, and more robust and active men."

Probably the most suitable fish for the consumptives to use are the white fish and trout, they contain but little fat, and are easily digested. To those who are called upon to put forth great nervous energy we would recommend fish once a day for supper. We would especially recommend the smoked halibut. "*Salmon* stands pre-eminent as a delicacy, and more nearly resembles meat than any other fish; fat is intermixed with the muscular fibre and underlies the skin, particularly of the abdomen; it is, therefore, rich, too rich for most invalids. *Mackerel, Herring, Pilchard, Sprat* and *Eel* are also fatty in their composition. These are less suitable than the white fish, for those whose powers of digestion are feeble. These are *Whiting, Sole, Haddock, Flounder, Cod, Turbot, Brill,* etc. Their flesh contains but little fat, except in the liver. *Whiting,* the chicken of fish, is the most delicate and easy to digest. *Sole* possesses the same excellencies and deserves it's popularity in the sick room. *Haddock* is firm, not so delicate, nor so digestible. *Flounder* is tasteless, but otherwise suitable. *Cod* is close, firm, tough, and indigestible by a weak stomach. *Turbot* has a richer flavor, but does not stand high as a food for invalids."

"The quality of all fish is superior before the spawning, when it is 'in season'" "Fish caught from deep seas are better than those from shallow bays. Fresh water fish from deep clear water, with stony bottom, are better than those from muddy shallows."

"For the invalid it should always be *boiled* or *broiled*, the fat added in *frying* renders the fish less digestible. Dried, salted, smoked, or pickled fish should not be seen in the sickroom."—Dr. Ruddock.

As a rule, *Shell fish* are unsuitable for the invalid, such as the *Lobster, Crab, Prawn and Shrimp*. They produce gastric irritation, etc., however:

OYSTERS form an exception, they are not only nutritious, but easily digested, excepting the hard portion that is attached to the shell; that should not be eaten. They should be eaten raw and well masticated before swallowing.

MEAT, as an article of diet, will be of great value in this disease, such as beef, mutton, and all kinds of game, including the various kinds of *poultry*. These should be fresh and plainly cooked. All rich sauces, gravy, or stuffing, should be excluded. The diet should be often varied, by the introduction of fish, game and poultry, but butcher's meat, not overloaded with fat, should preponderate.

The use of raw meat, where there is great emaciation, has often been invaluable. The French mix raw meat with sugar, and it forms a palatable sweetmeat, much liked by children. The French also practice drinking fresh lamb's blood. We have no doubt that blood is really valuable, being so easily assimilated, but it seems so disgusting, we believe few patients could be induced to use it.

Fresh vegetables, and especially ripe fruits, should be used in abundance.

CLOTHING—Consumptive people are very susceptible to the process celled "catching cold," consequently, they should be warmly clothed, though not to such an extent as to produce much persiration, or diseased fat. The extremities, especially, should be kept warm, to prevent congestion of blood to the lungs. The under-clothing is the most important point to be attended to, which should be of flannel, lambs wool or silk, and should be worn the year round. In summer it neutralizes any variation of temperature, and prevents sudden cooling by evaporation. In the winter it prevents the loss of the vital warmth of the body. In the winter an addition of a chamois leather vest may be worn over the flannel. In summer, during the warmest weather, a cautious change to a thinner flannel of fine merino may be advisable. The circulation seems so easily chilled, he cannot be too cautious in cold weather, by wrapping up warmly in furs and rugs, and if these do not keep his feet warm, use the means of a warm brick or flask of hot water to warm the feet. To prevent chest injury from the exposure of cold, every consumptive person should have a waistcoat buttoned up to the chin, and should wear the beard long. Women should avoid low dresses, and have a shawl ready for protection at all times.

■■

COUGH

This being one of the most prominent symptoms of pulmonary phthisis, requires the most careful and critical attention of the physician. No one symptom causes the patient more anxiety of mind than cough, and it makes no difference whether it is due to an organic lesions of the respiratory organs, or nervous irritation, caused by the reflex action from some distant organ; the cough must be cured, or the patient will seek some other physician. We are, therefore, *compelled* to include under this symptom all kinds of cough, and in doing so we most gladly and gratefully avail ourselves of the *practical,* clinical hints given to us by Dr. B. Hirschel. He says:

"A cough is a short, resonant, more or less forcible, impulsive expiration, with a more or less narrowed glottis, occurring generally after a deeper and more powerful inspiration. The cause of the different tones usually depends on the vocal formation. Expirations and inspirations often alternate. A cough can be produced voluntarily and also directly from the spinal cord; generally it is a reflex action depending on conditions of the mucous membrane (inflammation, catarrh, collection of mucus, nervous excitement, foreign bodies, such as dust and the like) of the superior parts of the air passages, especially of the larynx, and very often of the thoracic organs (bronchi, lungs).

"Formerly a cough was looked upon as the most positive sign of a lung affection, but experience has taught us that it may be totally absent in such cases, even in pneumonia and tuberculosis. On the other hand a cough may be present in conditions that have no connection with the thoracic organs, viz., in many cerebral and spinal diseases, from an elongated uvula, from diseases of the heart, pharynx, œsophagus, stomach, uterus and intestinal canal, so that it may even *simulate* phthisis.

"Likewise mechanical influences, such as tumors, may produce a cough by pressing on the vagus, but as soon as there is a spot in the respiratory organs where the tissue has become destroyed, greatly compressed, paralyzed by exudations, has become callous, or the susceptibility has become deadened (Wunderlich), then the irritation which caused the cough vanishes.

"The individual kinds of cough accord pretty definitely with certain forms of disease, so that from it's tone, or kind, we can draw conclusions as to the seat and form of the disease. But we must be very prudent in thus drawing conclusions, so as not to be led into manifold and great mistakes. Thus we like to differentiate laryngeal, tracheal, bronchial and pulmonary coughs from their tone and depth, yet we cannot do this with certainty. From it's degree, from the periodicity of the attacks, some pretend to recognize, now a beginning tuberculosis, then a simple catarrh, or a pneumonia, or emphysema, or spasmodic cough, yet there is no certain criterion for all this. The most insignificant morbid process may cause a severe and exhausting kind of cough, such as is often the case in neuroses.

"Our judgment must depend on the *repetition* of the cough, as also on the fact of it's being by *day*, by *night;* on it's *intermissions*, which sometimes lasts for weeks, and on it's being *paroxysmal;* in as much as the *tone* depends more on the condition of the *larynx* than on that of the more deeply lying thoracic organs, so it will be evident that it cannot be made use of for diagnostic purposes.

"The kind of secretion is of very great importance. Dry, chronic coughs are always suspicious, unless they are purely nervous.

"The cough is dry at the commencement of the organic disease, and only gets moist when the secretions become moveable. If the secretion comes from far down, the condition is always more dangerous than when the cough is superficial, and if the secretion becomes continuous and yet affords no relief, and the strength begins to fial, then the prognosis is unfavorable. Such is the case in chronic bronchitis, in tubercular suffering, and pulmonary abscesses.

"For the physician treating a cough, no matter what school he may belong to, it is important that he distinguish—

"a. The seat and point of origin of the cough.

"Here we must see whether the cough has it's origin in the larynx, in the trachea, in the bronchi and it's ramifications, or in the lung itself; in the pleura, in the heart, in the vagus, in the spinal cord—whether the mucous membrane or the parenchyma itself, the blood vessels or the nerves (primarily or secondarily) are affected.

"b. It's character, as regards the casual morbid process.

"It is especially important to know whether the process is *catarrhal*, simple or complicated with fever, acute or chronic catarrhal; whether it be *inflammatory* (acute or chronic, simple or croupous); or whether it be *organic* (with textural changes or not); or whether it be of *nervous* origin, peripheral or central).

"Arranged in this manner, we find cough is the most important symptom in the following *forms* of disease:

"I. In *simple catarrh*, acute or chronic, and with or without fever, to wit:

"(a) Laryngeal catarrh.

"(b) Tracheal catarrh.

"(c) Bronchial catarrh.

"(d) Pulmonary catarrh.

"(e) A peculiar form of epidemic catarrh, such as influenza.

II. In *inflammations of the vocal and respiratory organs*, acute or chronic in form, to wit:

"a. Laryngitis, simple or croupous (angina membranacea), diphtheritic, aphthous, pustular, submucous inflammations, œdema glottitis, perichondritis, epiglottitis.

"b. Tracheitis.

"c. Bronchitis—simple, croupous, diphtheritic.

"d. Pneumonia—simple, croupous, intestinal or hypostatic.

III. With *organic metamorphosis of the vocal and respiratory organs*.

"a.b. Laryngeal deformities and neoplasmata, helcosis laryngis, tuberculosis, polypi, carcinoma, stricture, stenosis, formation of diverticula, fistula of the larynx and of the trachea.

"c.d. Tuberculosis (infiltrated and miliary), hæmorrhage from bronchi and lungs, bronchiectasis, pulmonary emphysema, insufficiency and atrophy, cirrhosis, carcinoma, and other neoplasmata, ossifications, apostemata, gangrene of bronchi and lungs, pneumothorax.

"Here we must further enumerate :

"e. Affections of the pleura which excite pulmonary cough, either sympathetically or mechanically, as hæmorrhages, serous and inflammatory exudations, tuberculosis pleuræ; and finally,

"f. Cardiac affections which, by obstructing the reflux, produce pulmonary hyperemia, and thus excite cough.

IV. In *neuroses.* These arise either as primary forms from irritation of the vocal and respiratory nerves, or secondarily from central irritation, to wit:

"a. Spastic, tickling, spasmodic coughs.

b. Pertussis (according to some a neurosis of the bronchi, according to others, an affection of the vagus).

c. As symptoms of a nervous stenosis of the glottis in children and adults.

d. As symptoms of bronchial asthma of the nervous kind, or

e. Angina pectoris, cardiac spasm. Finally,

f. As a collateral phenomena of a central affection in the spinal cord, spinal irritation (hysteria)."

"The physician has also the *essential peculiarities of the cough itself* to bring within his ken, if he intends to make a good choice of remedies."

"1. The tone of the cough.

2. The subjective sensation, the kind of pain.

3. The seat, the origin as far as the patient can define it, or the tone and depth which it gives.

4. The repetition, time of occurrence.

5. The dryness, or the sputum, and it's nature.

6. The exacerbation or amelioration by certain conditions,

such as eating, drinking, lying down, moving about, rest, air, cold, warm, etc.

7. The concomitant phenomena, as fever, pains in other parts, complications."

"Under these forms we believe we have exhausted all the kinds of cough which present themselves for clinical treatment. A more elaborate description, which may be found in all the hand-books of pathology, our readers will willingly spare us, as such is not the object of this treatise which has more especially to deal with therapeutics."

Every case of cough we are called upon to attend, may vary at different hours, being sometimes dry and sometimes moist, but each one as a whole is either *predominantly dry or predominantly moist*.

1. Predominantly Dry

Aconite,	Dry,	aggravated	at night and by warmth.
Ambra,	"	"	in evening, relieved by open air.
Arnica,	"	"	day and night.
Arsenicum,	"	"	by cold air and at night.
Argentum,	"	"	in daytime.
Atropine,	"	"	day and night.
Bromine,	"	"	during daytime.
Bryonia,	"	"	at night, cold air and motion.
Causticum,	"	"	in evening and by getting warm.
Chamomilla	"	"	at night and by cold air.
Conium	"	"	at night, when lying down, and by deep inspirations.
Coffea,	"	"	at night.

COUGH

Cuprum,	Dry,	aggravated	day and night, and by cold damp air.
Drosera,	"	"	in the evening, after lying down, especially after midnight.
Dulcamara,	"	"	by damp cold air and getting wet.
Ferrum,	"	"	by cold air, and in the evening in bed.
Gelsemium,	"	"	at night.
Hyoscyamus,	"	"	at night, especially by lying down.
Ignatia,	"	"	by cold air, mental affections, motion and contact.
Iodium,	"	"	by going up stairs, and warm air.
Kali carb.,	"	"	by cold, damp air and at night.
Kali iod.,	"	"	by rest and damp weather.
Lachesis,	"	"	by sleep, at night; cold, damp weather, and touching the larynx.
Merc. sol,	"	"	at night; by heat and damp, cool air.
Nitric acid.,	"	"	at night; by damp, cool air and getting wet.
Nux vom.,	"	"	at 3 A. M., early in the morning; by getting cold and motion.
Opium,	"	"	especially at night, and by stimulants.

Phosphorus,	Dry,	aggravated	day and night; by change of weather, and cold air.
Rhus tox.,	"	"	by cold, damp atmosphere, getting wet and at night.
Rumex crispus,	"	"	by inhaling cold air and lying down at night.
Sepia,	"	"	all day, until midnight; by cold, damp east winds.
Spongia	"	"	at night; by cold, damp east winds, and with the head low.

2. Predominantly Moist

Amm. mur.,	Moist,	aggravations,	mornings, and by cold, damp weather.
Arsenate of Soda,	"	"	day.
Antimonium crud.,	"	"	mornings and by a warm atmosphere.
Aurum mur.,	"	"	morning and by cold air.
Calc. carb.,	"	"	by damp, cold weather.
Carbo veg.,	"	"	by damp, cold weather and evenings.
Carbo an.,	"	"	evenings and night, and by damp cold weather.
China,	"	"	intermittent and at night.
Chelidonium,	"	"	morning.
Digitalis,	"	"	from warmth.

COUGH

Hepar sulph.,	Moist,	aggravations,	night, by cold, or cold northeast wind.
Ipecacuanha,	"	"	by warm air, night and morning.
Kali bi.,	"	"	after eating; by awaking and deep inspirations.
Kali brom.,	"	"	at night.
Kreosote,	"	"	by cold air, morning and evening.
Lycoodium,	"	"	by cold, high winds evening and midnight.
Mercurius iod.,"		"	at night in a warm room; relieved by cold air.
Pulsatilla,	"	"	in a warm, close room; evenings, relieved by cool fresh air.
Sanguinaria,	"	"	evening and night, especially when lying down.
Senega,	"	"	by warm air; evenings and night, better in cool air.
Silicea,	"	"	by cold air, even the slightest draft, and at night.
Stannum,	"	"	by rapid motion, and at night.
Sulphur,	"	"	by cold or cold, damp weather, afternoon till midnight.

Tartar emetic, Moist, aggravation   in damp, cold weather
                                    and evenings.
Veratrum alb.,   ”   ”   from cold to warm air,
                                    by damp cold weather;
                                    by eating ice cream.

3. According to the Seat of the Cough, Affections of the Larynx and Trachea

Acon.,	Chel.,	Kali bi.,	Nux v.,
Bell.,	Coffea,	Kali iod.,	Opium,
Brom.,	Dig.,	Kali br.,	Phos.,
Bry.,	Dros.,	Lach.,	Puls.,
Conium,	Gels.,	Laur.,	Rumx.,
Cham.,	Hepar s.,	Merc. iod.,	Sang.,
Calc. i.,	Hyos.,	Merc. c.,	Silicea,
Carbo ac.,	Ipecac,	Merc.,	Sulph. and
Carbo v.,	Iodine,	Morphine,	Tartar emetic.
Caust.,	Ignatia,	Nitric acid,	

4. Affections of the Bronchi and Lungs

Acon.,	Cor. r.,	Kali c.,	Sulphur,
Ant. t.,	Dig.,	Kali br.,	Sang.,
Ars.,	Dros.,	Kreosote.,	Sars.,
Bell.,	Elaps,	Lyc.,	Silicea,
Bryonia,	Ferrum,	Merc.,	Stannum,
Calc.,	Hepar sulph.,	Phos.,	Tartar emetic,
Calc. ph.,	Ipecac,	Puls.,	Veratrum alb.
Carbo v.,	Iodine,	Rhus tox.,	and
Carbo an.,	Kali bi.,	Senega,	Verat. v.
Cuprum,	Kali iod,	Sepia,	

5. Stomach and Intestinal Canal

Sympathetic or reflex coughs usually call for a cerebrospinal remedy, such as:

Ant. c.,	Digitaline,	Lyc.,	Robinia,
Ant. t.,	Eupatorium,	Mercury,	Sang.,
Ars.,	Hepar sulph.,	Nux v.,	Sulphur and
Chel.,	Ipecac,	Puls.,	Veratrum alb.
Chin.,	Kali bi.,	Phos.,	
Carbo veg.,	Kreosote,	Podo.,	
Chamomilla,	Lachesis,	Quinine,	

6. Coughs from cerebral irritation especially call for the cerebral-centrics, like Bell.

7. Reflex cough from ovario-uterine irritation almost always demands cerebro-spinal remedies.

8. Heart and large blood vessels, (reflex cough) call for remedies such as:

Acon.,	Coll.,	Opium,	Spig.,
Ars.,	Dig.,	Iodine,	Sec.,
Bell.,	Digitaline,	Phos.,	Sulph., and
Cact.,	Laur.,	Spong.,	Verat. v.

9. Cough from acute inflammation: First stages must be combated with a cerebro-spinal remedy; second and third stage with organics.

10. Coughs from influenza or whooping cough, are mostly always cured with cerebro-spinal remedies.

11. Croupy cough, demands at first such remedies as Acon., Rhus v.; second stage, Spongia, Hepar, Iodine, Kali. bi., &c.

12. Croup : The acute stage demands a cerebro-spinal, the sub-acute and membranous forms are more successfully treated with the organic remedies.

Ulcerations, disorganizations, pseudoplasmata demand organic remedies.

13. Asthmatic, Suffocative Cough

Ars.,	Dros.,	Kreosotum,	Sulph.,
Asaf.,	Dig.,	Lach.,	Spong.,
Bell.,	Gels.,	Lyc.,	Sep.,
Cham.,	Hyos.,	Nux v.,	Tartar emetic.,
Caust.,	Ipecac,	Opium,	Verat. alb.,
Carbo v.,	Iodium,	Morphine,	Verat. v.
Cupr.,	Kali iod.,	Puls.,	
Chin.,	Kali bi.,	Phos.,	

14. Morning Cough

Acon.,	Chin.,	Kreos.,	Staph.,
Alum,	Cina,	Nat. m.,	Stram.,
Atropine,	Dig.,	Nux v.,	Verat. alb.
Caust.,	Iod.,	Phos. ac.,	
Chel.,	Ipecac,	Squill.,	

15. Evening Cough

All. c.,	China,	Mez.,	Sang.,
Ambr.,	Cina,	Mosch.,	Seneg.,
Ars.,	Dros.,	Morphine,	Sep.,
Atropine,	Eup. per.,	Mur. ac.,	Sil.,
Bar. c.,	Ferr.,	Nat. m.,	Spong.,

COUGH

Bell., Hep.,   Nit. ac.,   Stann.,
Bry.,   Ign.,   Phos.,   Stict,
Calc., Lach.,   Phos. ac.,   Sulph.,
Carbo an., Lyc.,   Puls.,   Sul. ac.,
Carbo v., Magn. m., Rhus t.,   Verat. alb. and
Caust., Merc.,   Rumx.,   Zinc.

16. Night Cough

Acon., Bry.,   Cor. r.,   Merc.,
Alum,   Calc.,   Dulc.,   Phos.,
Ambr., Carbo an., Hyos.,   Rumx.,
Anac., Cham.,   Ipecac,   Sang.,
Ant. t., Cocc.,   Kali c.,   Seneg.,
Ars.,   Cact.,   Kali bi.,   Sil. and
Bell., Con.,   Magn.,   Verat.

17. After Midnight

Acon., Chin.,   Hyos.,   Nux v.,
Bell., Dros.,   Kali,   Samb.

We will now endeavor to give the special indications of each remedy in an alphabetical order. My best guide to the selection of a remedy is the nature of the cough, for you are all well aware that every cough is either predominantly loose or predominantly dry. This is my first inquiry; and my second is to know the nature of the expectoration; the third, the time of day, or night, and the fourth, the concomitant symptoms.

ACONITUM NAPELLUS (DRY) — Dry croupy cough, resulting from an exposure to dry cold air, short, dry, titillating cough, and every inspiration seems to increase the cough. The patient is greatly disturbed in his sleep by the cough, and as soon as he is fairly settled down to sleep again, the cough recommences, and so continually repeats itself. Uncontrollable anguish with great fear of death. Sudden inflammation with high fever, great restlessness from exposure, whereby the perspiration is suddenly suppressed. Dry, tickling, night cough, in a restless, feverish patient; cough with active hæmorrhages, and great fear of death.

This remedy is especially adapted to people of a sanguine temperament and a full, plethoric habit, where the primary or inflammatory stage has not passed. If high fever is present, it suits both a loose, as well as a dry cough; but as a rule, it acts best where there is a dry cough, aggravated at night.

"There is most always a tingling sensation in the chest after coughing. There may be stitches in the chest and side, which are often severe enough to interfere considerably with respiration, can only get half inch respirations; sometimes there is an oppression of the chest, without pain, which keeps one from taking a deep breath, palpitations of the heart, with great anguish." In dry bronchial catarrh, in its most obstinate form, it is the most reliable agent we have. It is also of great value in these long fits of dry morning and evening coughs, so trying to the patient from their everyday recurrence.

"Where the left lung is most involved, and the pleura is at the same time implicated, manifested by a sharp stitching pain on breathing, the cough which would be very hard were it not suppressed on account of the pain, is almost dry, it being extremely difficult to raise anything. The little that is brought up is *tenacious,* falling in a round lump, and of a dark cherry red color. "Aconite 30 is assuredly the remedy."

— C. PEARSON, M.D.

Aconite cough is aggravated in the evening, and more particularly at night and in a warm room.

Amelioration in the open air and when still.

AMBRA GRISEA (DRY) — Ambra cough has its seat in the spinal marrow or indirectly in the uterine system, and is purely nervous, originating in the nervous spinal centre. Hysterical women, with a constant hacking cough, scraping and copious expectoration. Lean delicate, sickly looking people.

Highly hysterical women, cough with expectoration of grayish mucus, and abundant eructations.

Reflex cough, from spinal or ovario-uterine irritation, and not from any organic lesions of the respiratory organs. Worse evenings and better in the open air.

AMMONIUM MURIATICUM (MOIST) — Chronic catarrh in old people, with bronchiectasis, emphysema of the lungs with profuse, thick, whitish expectoration, the cough sounds much looser than it is; much mucoid rattling without expectoration. Fat, bloated and lax individuals who are indolent and sluggish.

The ammonia cough is aggravated in the morning and frequently accompanied with sobbing and hiccough. Speaking of Amm. carb., Dr. Meyhoffer says: "We have found it of great use in very chronic cases of copious bronchial secretions, great difficulty in expectoration, and bronchial dilation. Low vitality and atony of the bronchial surface are leading indications. The hand and the ear will detect numerous coarse rattles, and yet the patient experiences no necessity to clear his chest of its morbid production, cachectic conditions and old age are its great indices. The second and third dilutions act unexceptionally." The cough is worse in cold, wet weather.

> **ARNICA MONTANA (DRY)** — Cough resulting from the bad effects of mechanical injuries; bruised sensation in any part of the body; inflammation of the skin and cellular tissue, with extreme tenderness on pressure. The bed on which he lies feels too hard, keeps changing position from place to place.

For some unknown reason to me, our school hardly, if ever, prescribes Arnica for coughs, although it ought to be very valuable in a cough that is predominantly dry and worse at nights, especially if brought on from mechanical injuries accompanied with much myalgia of the intercostal muscles. In organic cough, where serous exudation has taken place; dry cough and hoarseness from over exertion; dry concussive cough, with difficult or bloody expectoration, etc., etc.

> **ANTIMONIUM CRUDUM (MOIST)** — Thick, milky white coating on the tongue; mucous membranes are loaded with mucus, with slow digestion; nausea and vomiting; reflex cough from the stomach or abdomen; great emaciation, with excessive grief; eating, ever so little, produces obstinate vomiting; aged people, with corns, horny excrescences, and inflammation of the skin; aversion to washing.

This is a splendid cough remedy, where the cough is predominantly loose, and seems to have its starting point from irritation of the mucous membrane in the stomach with much vomiting, diarrhea and a heavily coated tongue. Its great centre of action is upon the filaments of the vagi that are distributed to the mucous membranes of the lungs and digestive organs, especially the stomach. Like Tartar emetic its action hardly ever goes on to inflammation. A tubercular

COUGH

cough will not be much benefitted by it; for simple bronchitis, after the second stage has commenced, with a loose cough, this is a first class remedy.

> ARSENCIUM ALBUM (DRY) — Cough that is predominantly dry, in organic diseases of an incurable and destructive nature; cough excited by a sensation as if the fumes of sulphur were inhaled; cough followed by an increased difficulty in breathing, great exhaustion, with severe dyspnea, and nightly aggravations, rapid and great prostration, with sinking of the vital forces; burning pains, parts burn like fire; pains greatly aggravated by rest, relieved by motion; extreme anguish and fear of death; cannot lie down for fear of suffocation; great thirst, drinks often, but little at a time. Lymphatic people that are sad and irritable.

Dr. Hirschel's description of the arsenicum cough is most graphic, and to the point. He says it "applies in all kinds of coughs; predominantly, however, in *dry cough*. In *spasmodic cough* it is indicated only in its typical form. *Whooping cough* does not lie in its range. It is indicated in *chronic affections* of a torpid or dangerous nature, and in acute cases of the same nature, especially indicated for cough in organic diseases of an incurable or destructive nature, either in the larynx, bronchi, lungs, pleura or heart; its choice depends upon others than cough symptoms. These functional symptoms are: dyspnea, asthma, suffocative spells, cyanosis, heart symptoms of all kinds, disturbed circulation, decomposition of blood, exudations, decay and gangrene of organic substances, disorganizations, and excessive pains. *Constitutional* indications are : exhaustion of life-power, collapse, high degree of weakness, syncope, anæmia, nervous irritability, disposition to ulceration, hydræmia and the like. *Conditions* are : typical forms, nightly aggravations, worse from lying down, drinking and change of weather." I cannot state anything more practical and to the point, in the use of this remedy in cough than is given by J.Meyhoffer, M.D., in his work on "Chronic Diseases of the Organs of Respiration." He says: "*Arsenicum* is, after Aconite, one of the most important medicines in *dry catarrh* not of recent date. It operates its most striking effects in the form of dyspnea, which results from a more or less extensive emphysema and consecutive pulmonary congestion. Thus the difficulty of breathing which is relieved by Ars. does not entirely cease in the intervals of coughing, and also returns in periodical, severe paroxysms, especially during the night. None the less remarkable is its action when the obstruction in the pulmonary circulation is caused by regurgitation of the blood from the ventricles into the auricles. There may be œdema of the lungs, but the bronchial secretion is scanty, and a sensation of dryness in the respiratory lining prevails. The patients complain of an exasperating titillation in the windpipe or under the sternum, chiefly at night, that provokes a dry, wheezing, often a very violent cough; this is attended, after a time, by a white, frothy, sometimes sticky mucous. Its action is prompt and intense, numberless invalids, who without its aid, would have passed agonizing nights, are, by its use, enabled to rest tranquilly. This vitalizing action of the mineral on the nervous system has often been the means of saving the lives of children who arrived at the last stage of a suffocative catarrh.

No remedy will be found more powerful or more sure to raise the vitality when asphyxia is too far advanced for the exhibition of Tartar emetic and the tumultuous agitation of the heart foretells its fast approaching paralysis.

Though rarely of much service in simple catarrh, Arsenicum is invaluable in the treatment of bronchitis connected with deficient assimilation and arrested organic metamorphosis. As a hæmatic and ganglionary neurotic it displays remarkable regulating effects on nutrition in great emaciation or tendency to fatty deposits; in anæmia, malaria, cachexia and fatty degeneration of the kidneys. It is less valuable in all forms of bronchitis dating from a herpetic taint."

In anæmic subjects, with dry, asthmatic, nightly cough, or if there is a disturbed circulation from atheromatous disease of the valves in the heart, Arsenicum will be found of much value. Anguish and despondency are prominent in cases that call for the use of Arsenicum.

ARSENATE OF SODA (MOIST) — Organic cases where the second stage has set in with a loose cough, night sweats and diarrhea.

Dr. Ruddock gives the following indications for this remedy: "Severe cough and profuse expectoration; hectic fever; night sweats; diarrhea. Even when auscultation detects abscesses in the lungs, the disease may sometimes be controlled by this remedy."

Aggravations, at night, after midnight, in cold air, or getting cold; after drinking; from exertion; while lying down with the head low; from cold drinks; always wants to be wrapped up warmly, and on going up stairs, relieved in lying with the head high; going down; from warm food or drinks, and near a stove.

ARGENTUM NITRICUM (DRY) — A withered and dried up person from disease. Patient can't think, can't walk, very dizzy; minutes seem hours to the patient; time seems so long that the patient worries about everything. Is in a great hurry to do things. Great distention of the stomach with gas. Fluids seem to run straight through the intestinal canal without stopping. Ulceration of the bowels with diarrhea.

This remedy has a special and specific action upon the cartilaginous system; in tuberculosis, with ulceration of the larynx and trachea, with dry, racking cough, this remedy will be of great service, especially if there is a syphilitic taint in the system.

Dr. J. Meyhoffer says : "Nitrate of silver proves a highly beneficial agent in all the stages of tuberculous laryngitis. In the beginning of the disease, when the throat and larynx are much inflamed, with titillation in the latter, much hawking or spasmodic cough and accumulation of phlegm in the throat. At a later period, when the edge of the ulcers are the seat of luxuriant granulations, the inhalations of the stronger solutions of this salt produce excellent effects, as they reduce the morbid growths. In several instances we have ascertained incipient serous infiltration of the sub-mucous tissue in the last stage of laryngeal phthisis, and seen it give way to these solutions. They have, however, the drawback of blackening the skin or linen with which they come in contact; that can only be partly avoided by inhaling the steam through a glass tube, or by otherwise protecting the exposed parts. Sometimes, therefore, when wishing to act with more energy, without employing the caustic in substance, we use insufflation into the larynx by a slightly curved glass tube, with one or two grains of the first decimal trituration of silver nitrate. The frequent effect is a violent fit of coughing, but the growth is thoroughly acted upon, and the operation need not be repeated more than three or four times. Should the vegetations be extensive, however, or in cauliflower form, or if by their situation they should cause dyspnea, they must either be destroyed by the *porte-caustique*, or removed with laryngeal scissors. The same operation is to be performed on the detached flaps of the mucous membrane; difficult and painful deglutition, with extensive ulceration of the epiglottis, is often only relieved by the direct application of the caustic.

"We use *Argentum nitricum,* in all it's preparations; from the second and third potency, to be the local application of the lunar caustic, and from one to six grains to an ounce of water for inhalations.

"We have seen this mineral master inflammation and swelling of the posterior wall and lining of the larynx, attended by a sensation in the vocal organs, with hoarseness or loss of voice, continued or vain efforts to swallow, pain and soreness in deglutition, and hawking, considerable mucopurulent expectoration, titillation in the larynx, with a dry spasmodic cough. The third to the twelfth attenuations."

AURUM MURIATICUM (MOIST) — Suicidal monomania, accompanied with extreme depression of spirits; dread of some impending calamity, unrefreshing sleep, loss of ambition and energy; disposition to dwell upon some imaginary ailments, diminution of verile strength, great difficulty of breathing during the night, violent palpitations of the heart; nightly bone pains; ozæna.

Acts decidedly upon the lymphatic glandular system, much like mercury, and is adapted to suffocative coughs that are inclined to be loose, in scrofulous subjects, especially if they have chronic nasal catarrh, with ulceration of the nasal bones; so if the patient has been abused with mercury, or has the effects of syphilis grafted upon him, with nightly bone pains, Aurum greatly resembles Arsenicum and Silicea. Suffocative cough with palpitations of the heart, and extreme despondency.

"I have had cases of a dry spasmodic (or what I should call nervous) cough, peculiar to females, generally periodical, every night, commencing at sunset, and continuing through the night, going off with the rising of the sun, and freedom from it during the day. Aurum 200 cures every time. In the plain text, cough for want of breath at night." L. B. Wells, M. D.

Aggravation in the morning, in the cold air, on getting cold; better from moving, and in the warm air. It's action is similar to that of Iodide of Potash. As an inter-current, where the Iodide has ceased to act, Aurum muriaticum, will be of a great value.

> **BELLADONNA (DRY)** — Pains come and go with great celerity. Furious delirium, wild look, wishes to strike, bite or quarrel. Face flushed, eyes red, rage, tears, bites, and shrieks; violent congestion of blood to the head, with a strong throbbing of carotids. Throbbing headache worse from motion and noise is intolerable. Eyes red and glistening; photophobia; great dryness of the mouth and fauces; tonsils bright red and swollen, spasms of the throat; symptoms worse evenings and at night.

The primary or starting point of the affection is in the brain. A hard, dry, teasing, spasmodic cough predominates, generally accompanied with inflammation of the throat, and difficult, painful deglutition. Dr. Hirschel says that Bell. has "great sensitiveness, in contradistinction to the irritable Aconite. Vasomotory stimulation with increased nervosity. The chief remedy, therefore, for sensitive persons, women and children; for erethic inflammatory forms, not for croupy, plastic ones, for spastic states, *cough dry, barking, spasmodic, in paroxysms,* with titillation in the trachea or bronchi; *aggravation at night,* and when continuous, sensation as of having swallowed dust; *amelioration from anything cold,* sensation of constriction in throat, difficulty in swallowing; congestion of the head; stitches in the chest. In simple catarrhs, in inflammatory forms with a catarrhal character (larynx, trachea down to the lungs), specially in the first stage, more in bronchitis, especially in pneumonia, in the beginning of whooping cough; influenza; in affections of the brain, spinal cord or heart; inflammation of parts adjacent to the respiratory organs. In stenosis of the glottis, in bronchial asthma, as an intercurrent remedy

COUGH

in chronic cases. Examination of the affected parts shows a pinkish, smooth redness in the pharynx, uvula and fauces." Baehr says : "A disposition to perspire while the skin is very hot, with a dry, continuous, distressing, spasmodic cough; short paroxysms of cough but very violent, especially towards evening, no expectoration, or else a yellowish, tenacious, blood streaked, scanty expectoration. Sensation of great fulness in the lungs without pain." Larynx exceedingly painful, with constriction of the trachea, hoarseness, paralytic aphonia of a cerebro-spinal origin, that has come on very suddenly. As soon as the cough commences to loosen up, the usefulness of Belladonna passes and another remedy must be selected.

Aggravation in the afternoon, at night and by moving or touching the parts.

Ameliorated, while reposing.

ATROPINUM (DRY) — This is a precious remedy for cough, but it's true characteristics are not yet known with the precision enough to separate them from those of Belladonna. All the symptoms, are the same, excepting the vascular symptoms; the congestions and inflammations of Belladonna do not appear so prominently in the Atropine cough, but the *neurotic elements predominate*. This neurotic element seems to predominate in all diseases where Atropine acts better than Belladonna, the parts seem to be in a nervous, irritable state instead of a congested inflammatory condition. Many cases of cough have yielded most beautifully and rapidly under the influence of Atropine after Belladonna, which though indicated, had failed to entirely cure. In my opinion Atropine is of much more service to us in a dry, hard, tearing cough than Belladonna, and ought to be employed much more frequently. I use the third decimal dissolved in water.

> **BROMIUM (DRY)** — Croupy, dry, rough, barking or whistling cough. Tickling in the throat as if from sulphur vapour; sensation of coldness in the larynx; for blondes rather than for persons having a white, delicate skin. Has a remarkable action upon the glandular system, and respiratory organs.

This remedy has not been given very often in cough, and it's true sphere is not yet fully known. Dry cough, with suffocation, seems to be it's indication but Prof. Guernsey says, "with the croupy sound there is a good deal of loose rattling in the larynx during breathing and coughing, *but there is no choking during cough as there is in* Hepar." In my opinion, Dr. Hirschel is correct when he says Bromine is indicated "for swelling and hypertrophy of the mucous membrane (Iodine for the exudation), of the upper parts of the respiratory organs, of a catarrhal, inflammatory or organic origin; dry, croupy cough, with scraping titillation and hoarseness, small follicles are found on the posterior mucous membrane of the pharynx, extending from there to the larynx and producing continued titillating cough. The larynx is painful on touch. Anatomically, we might say *Spongia* is more suitable for stasis, simple inflammation; *Bromine* for swelling and hypertrophy of the mucous membranes; *Iodine* for exudation.

Aggravation of cough during day time.

> **BRYONIA ALBA (DRY)** — Symptoms greatly aggravated by motion. Patient cannot sit up; lips dry and cracked; cannot sit up from nausea and faintness; everything tastes bitter. Diarrhea from hot weather, or constipation, stools hard and dry as if burnt; irritable headache as if it would burst open.

Bryonia's great sphere of usefulness is found in inflammatory affections of the respiratory organs, the lungs and their enveloping membranes, that have advanced to the stage of effusion, Dr. Hirschel says : "Bryonia stands in close relation to the chest. It frequently follows Aconite, to remove the debris, and is therefore in a certain way more powerful than Aconite, which acts more on the general state and less on the local, and *vice versa* in comparison to Mercurius, the latter acting more on the local state, whereas Bryonia affects the general state; Bryonia brings on *resolution* in catarrhs, resorption in inflammation; is chiefly indicated in the second stage for slightly plastic but not highly graded inflammatory forms in croup. It is the chief remedy in bronchial affections (therefore in influenza); in catarrhal pneumonia only applicable where hepatization passes over in resolution, or where the pleura is at the same time affected, perhaps also in chronic pneumonia. The Bryonia cough is concussive by coming dry from the sternal region, as if the chest would burst, with scanty yellow, or blood streaked thin mucus, frequently with vomiturition and vomiting, especially after eating, with status gastricus, difficulty of breathing, pleuritic stitches, muscular pains, sensation of soreness in the throat and below it." Dr. W. H. Holcomb says: "Bryonia for a dry, concussive cough, producing pain both in the head and chest, with characteristic stitching pains." Dr. Guernsey says : "Bryonia cough is at night in bed, *compelling* one to *spring up* and *assume an erect posture at once*. This seems an involuntary motion." A prominent indication for this remedy is rheumatic and bruising pains in the muscles of the chest and back. Dr. Baehr says; "We wish to state, as an evidence of the healing powers of this drug that we scarcely ever notice under it's administration a copious secretion of the so called sputa cocta, and that the resorption of the infiltration takes place with very little, or perhaps without any expectoration, or, judging from the stand point of pathology, taking place in it's most perfect form." This is practical knowledge. "Where the cough and fever are very similar to those of Aconite, except that there being much less inflammation in the pleura and consequently less pain, the patient is enabled to cough much harder, raising, however, but little, which is tough, falling in round jelly like lumps, but in colour, *is much lighter, almost a yellow or soft brick shade*, Bryonia 30 or 200 will scarcely fail to cure nine cases out of every ten." C. Pearson, M. D.

Aggravation, in the evening and night; from cold air and motion.

> **CALCAREA CARBONICA (MOIST)** — Constitutional diseases of scrofulous people, with a leucophlegmatic temperament; prone to affections of the mucous membranes, imperfect assimilation of food to tissue. Dry and flabby skin; children with large open fontanelles, and much perspiration in drops on the head, which wets the pillow far around, during sleep. Excessive debility; walking produces great fatigue; while going up stairs, is out of breath and has to sit down; feet feel as if they had cold, damp stockings on; cold continually; women who menstruate profusely and too often; great emaciation, with a constant disposition to take cold.

This is one of the best and most useful remedies in the *materia medica* for consumption. It acts with great power, through the ganglionic system upon the *lymphatics, mucous membranes, skin and osseous tissue,* and we find it especially useful in diseases and individualities in whom the process of formation and reformation is imperfectly performed, as in childhood during dentition, rachitis and in lymphatic constitutions. It is one of the most useful cough remedies we have, and it is adapted more especially to a loose cough, acts well in either a dry or loose cough, many physicians claim that a dry cough is it's forte, but with me, after a cough has lasted a while and has passed, or is passing, into a loose, moist cough, Calcarea is our chief remedy in scrofulosis and tuberculosis, and therefore beneficial in many chronic coughs, especially in ulcerative processes of the larynx or in other kinds of cough resting on an organic base." Marcy and Hunt say : "Persons curable by it are of a lymphatic temperament, scrofulous, or rickety; show plethora of the veins, easily take cold, are frail, poorly fed, but tend to grow fat. It's application in consumption is chiefly restricted to cases in which these features predominate. The patient is feeble in body and mind, though in some cases mentally precocious, and often regarded as a genius; he is subject to depression of spirits, weeping mood; restless and anxious; has no hope of recovery, is hypochondriacal; hair falls off, eyes are feeble, cannot bear gas light; and he suffers from all possible derangements of digestion; the nervous system becomes excessively irritable, especially in females, hysteria, fault finding, nervous exhaustion, especially menorrhagia; in males spermatorrhea or exhausting emissions. It is proper in the stage of purulent expectoration, especially after sulphur or nitric acid."

Dr. Meyhoffer says: "We fully agree with Baehr, who indicates emphysematous catarrh as being especially within it's sphere of action, no less commendable is this mineral in bronchial dilatation and putrid expectoration."

Dr. Holcomb says, "Calcarea carb. frequently softens and mitigates a harsh, dry, recent cough, but has quite a different indication in serious, chronic and organic bronchial disease." This is one of our most powerful constitutional drugs," which frequently finds it's indications in the general symptoms or constitution of the patient, quite as prominently as in the specific symptoms of an individual case, and yet characteristic symptoms are not by any means wanting; the cough is almost always accompained with a more or less profuse expectoration, early *putting on a purulent character*. Amelioration from lying upon the back; aggravation from lying upon the sides. Calcarea, with us, has shown a more marked control over the upper half of the right lung than over any other portion of either lung."

Dr. C. Dunham says : "Short, spasmodic cough, in brief, but frequently repeated paroxysms; excited by a tickling, as if from feathers or down in the throat and trachea, in the *evening* and *night, without* expectoration, but in the morning and during the day attended by copious mucous or purulent, yellow expectoration and is sometimes bloody, having generally a sour taste and an offensive odor."

Aggravation, in damp, cold atmosphere, from getting wet; from drinking, talking, lying down and during sleep; relieved in dry, warm weather.

CARBO VEGETABILIS (MOIST) — Great foulness of the secretions, patient wants more air, wants to be fanned all the time. The most innocent food disagrees. Excessive accumulation of gas in the stomach and bowels, the gas is generated by the walls of the viscera, rather than from the fermentation of food, much bleeding of the gums; when eating or drinking, sensation as if the stomach or abdomen would burst. Icy coldness of the parts with a livid, purple look; hippocratic face with cold breath, and general coldness of the whole body. Long lasting hoarseness.

Diseases of the lungs, where there is a great tendency of the chest to perspire and the patient takes cold with the least change of temperature. The Carbo v. cough is moist and loose in patients that have become greatly enfeebled by long lasting diseases; the expectoration is copious, yellow, greenish and very fetid, accompanied with an extremely fetid breath. Baehr says: "Cough in old people, with emphysema and hypertrophy of the lungs, heart and abdominal viscera are very much impeded, very sensitive to cold, worse at night, expectoration profuse, especially if the larynx is invaded. "Dr. Reis says : "*Chronic catarrh of the bronchi and stomach.* Cough with copious expectoration at night and in the morning; tightness of the chest; sickly appearance, great sleeplessness at night, through the day pyrosis, with a great flow of water from the mouth." Dr. Guernsey says: "Respiration oppressed; having some kind of bad smell; quick cough with expectoration in the morning and no expectoration in the evening; neglected pneumonia, with expectoration of a dirty yellow colour, and smelling badly." Dr. Meyhoffer says "*Carbo v.* is the panacea for poor, exhausted constitutions and aged people with great torpor of the bronchial lining, profuse muco-purulent sputa, or deficient power of expectoration with symptoms of imperfect oxidation of blood; lips and nails blue, extremities cold. The weaker the invalids, the better the higher dilutions work."

Dr. C. C. Smith says: "Frequent and *easy epistaxis*, generally worse at *night*, or in the *forenoon*, followed by *pain* over the chest, and a pale face; sensitiveness to sudden changes of temperature; *hoarsness* towards *evening*, about 5 o'clock; pains in the chest burning." Carbo v. is more strongly indicated if the larynx is involved. The patient is so greatly reduced, and the lugs so much involved, the remedy must not be expected to act immediately.

Aggravations in the evening till midnight; by walking in open air, especially in damp, cold air, by passing from a warm into a cold atmosphere; by becoming cold, and by eating or drinking cold food or liquids, by butter or fat food and in the morning.

CARBO ANIMALIS (MOIST) — Scrofulous, venous constitutions, with enlarged glands, great debility, and a great disposition to perspire around the thorax. Great disposition to take cold, patient feels completely exhausted, can hardly stand, if it is a woman, menstruation exhausts her, so that she can hardly speak. Earthy coloured face, copper coloured spots on the face and body, secretions acrid.

Cirrhotic dyscrasia with swelling and ulceration of the glands. This remedy is adapted to chronic coughs after they have reached the second or suppurative stage; the cough is loose and rattling, expectoration profuse of thick, yellow, greenish, fetid sputa, with much fetor of breath, accompanied with debilitating, profuse, night sweats. The constitution of the patient will have much to do in the selection of this remedy, if the patient has inveterate and obstinate indurations of the glands; the complexion is of a coppery colour, and the disease is well advanced, the remedy will be found of great utility. It's indications greatly resemble those of *Carbo v.*

Aggravation of the cough in damp, cold air and at night.

CAUSTICUM (DRY) — Scrofulous people with yellow complexions. Cannot keep the upper eyelids up, they are nearly paralyzed, and will fall down over the eyes, great melancholy, looks on the dark side of everything. Constant sensation as if lime was being burned in the stomach, with flatulence and waterbrash. Catarrhal aphonia. Dry hard cough with involuntary emissions of urine. This is the clergymen's remedy for hoarsness and loss of voice from over-exertion. Inability to expectorate.

This is a remedy of great value in the treatment of diseases of the respiratory organs. The great predominating symptom is a dry hoarse cough, with aphonia; for complete aphonia no remedy can equal it. If the cough is loose, the patient is obliged to swallow what is raised, cannot spit it out. Involuntary passing of urine during a fit of coughing is a valuable indication, especially if there is an excessive amount of uric acid in the urine. Chronic morning hoarseness, with dry cough and much congestion of the fauces; catarrhal aphonia, weakness of the voice from over exertion, phlegm in the throat that cannot be hawked up, which produces nausea. Hard, dry, racking, hoarse, morning cough, with involuntary emissions of urine. "Dry, hollow cough, with soreness in the chest, caused by tickling and mucus in the throat, with expectoration only at night, of an acrid tasting mucus, which

COUGH

he cannot raise but has to swallow again." — *Jahr.* Dr. Guernsey says : "Cough, after getting *warm* in *bed,* or after recovering the *natural warmth* from a colder state, cough relieved by a cold drink; spirting of urine with the cough." The larynx seems to the center for the action of Causticum, not withstanding it also affects all the respiratory organs.

Cough is aggravated in the evening, and by getting warm. Relieved by cold air, or taking a cold drink of water and in damp weather.

CHAMOMILLA (DRY) — Extremely impatient, cannot answer one civilly; pain makes him furious, and is out of patience with everybody; child is excessively fretful; must be carried all the time to keep him quiet; headstrong, even unto quarrelling; extremely sensitive to pain; one cheek red and the other pale; severe flatulent colic, abdomen distended like a drum; green watery diarrhea, or like chopped eggs and spinach; nightly diarrhea with severe colic, in children.

Through the cerebro-spinal system, Chamomilla acts upon the respiratory organs, producing a dry suffocative cough, that generally is worse at night and in children during sleep. The predominating cough of Chamomilla is a dry, scraping cough, with a snappish, ugly disposition.

Dr. Hirschel says : "*Chamomilla* is a grand anti-spasmodic, especially in women and children. The picture of nervous bronchial asthma is beautifully given in the symptoms; suffocative constriction of the chest, as if the throat was throttled with a constant desire to cough." In the first stages of cough in children, with over sensitiveness of the nerves, this remedy exerts a happy influence.

Aggravations at night, by anger, cold air, especially a dry east and north wind.

Relieved by becoming warm and from warm drinks.

> **CHINA (MOIST)** — The system has been debilitated by the loss of vital fluids, as blood, semen, diarrhea, over lactation, night sweats and leucorrhea; symptoms aggravated every other day. The symptoms are aggravated by the slightest contact; moving or touching the parts brings on intolerable neuralgia; long lasting, congestive headache, with singing and roaring in the ears; enormous distention of the abdomen with gas; diarrhea of undigested food; debilitating night sweats; symptoms are intermittent.

This remedy is not what might be called a cough remedy, but for peculiar states of the system it becomes a remedy of great value; for instance, in cases where the vitality has sunk very low, with great debility, and the disease is very dilatory in character. Cough, when the head is *low*, it must be *raised;* violent cough after eating; cough with jelly like expectoration. Dr. Meyhoffer says : "China would be sadly missed, if not at hand in chronic bronchitis with loud coarse rattles, great debility and weakness; anæmic and œdematous swelling of the lower extremities. It is often the natural successor of Ars."

Baehr says : "China is indicated if the pulmonary affection seems to constitute the whole difficulty, but still more, if it commences with the symptoms of severe hyperemia of the liver, and if the patients very soon show a cachectic appearance. It is well known how often pains in the liver constitute symptoms of tuberculosis."

Marcy and Hunt say : "It not only prevents destruction of nerve tissue, but, by it's well known effects on the functions of nutrition, contributes greatly to the reparative process. It may, therefore, be regarded as the great conservator of the nervous system in conditions of febrile excitement or nervous prostration. Drs. Kidd and Gedham spoke most highly of the results they had obtained from the pure tincture of

China in the advanced stage of phthisis. The power of China and the Sulphate of quinine in arresting the destructive metamorphosis of tissue is only beginning to be appreciated." If the great symptom of exhaustion from loss of fluids be kept in mind, it will bring the use of China in the last stages of cough to hold up the patient.

Aggravations, in the evening, in damp, cold weather; from touching the parts; from eating and drinking and lying with the head low.

> **CHELIDONIUM MAJUS (MOIST)** — Constant pain under the lower inner angle of the right shoulder. Long continued cough with lungs filled with mucus; pneumonia of the right side, where there is a great deal of mucus. Many liver symptoms with cough.

This is a trump card for acute cases of cough, when lungs are filled with mucus, from paralysis of the vagi, accompanied with many bilious symptoms and great despondency; aggravation, early in the morning.

> **CONIUM MACULATUM (DRY)** — Sad, despondent people, great vertigo, particularly when lying down, and when turning over in bed. Much difficulty in voiding urine, it flows and stops again repeatedly during urination; in women there is great tenderness of the breasts preceding menstruation, very painful in walking or the least jar. Nocturnal, dry, hard, spasmodic cough, greatly aggravated by lying down. Yellow skin; cancerous, scrofulous people with indurated glands; cough with great irritation of the bladder.

This is one of our most valuable remedies in dry, teasing, spasmodic cough, lasting a long time after lying down at night. The Conium cough is always dry and greatly aggravated by light air. Dr. Hirschel says: "It's action takes in organic metamorphosis. It's cough is periodic, dry, caused by an itching, scraping titillation in the throat, or under the sternum; short convulsive cough, excited by a horizontal position, *speaking* or *laughing*. The two latter exciting causes of the cough are decisive for the choice of the remedy. The irritation of the cough is seated in the trachea or upper bronchi. In whooping cough it suits towards the end of the nervous stage, after Drosera, when speaking and laughing cause paroxysms, whose power and duration are already broken. In nervous, bronchial asthma it shows good effects and certainly brings alleviation in organic cases."

It's action on the laryngeal nerves and larynx is strongly marked in the provings, and has often been confirmed in practice; it's action on the lungs is less marked. The Conium cough is centred in the larynx, trachea and upper bronchi.

Aggravations, at night, when lying down; from deep inspirations, laughing, moving constantly, &c.

COFFEA (DRY) — Great nervous irritability; wakeful, and excitement of the intellect. Acute sensitive hearing. Great sleeplessness and nervous irritability. The pains are in supportable; cannot bear to be touched, the parts are so sensitive. All the senses greatly excited; affections after sudden emotions.

For reflex, dry, spasmodic coughs, Coffea will often be found useful, if it is accompanied with great nervous excitability. Continuous inclination to cough, with sensation of rawness in the trachea. Oppression of the chest; obliged to take short inspirations. Nightly cough, with great sleeplessness. Aggravations at night.

CUPRUM METALLICUM (DRY) — Cough, characterized by the long, uninterrupted continuance of it's paroxysms; trembles after coughing; relieved by drinking cold water. Strong metallic taste in the mouth. Drinking cold water relieves the cough.

Cuprum cough is of a suffocative, dry, spasmodic nature; long continued paroxysms of convulsive coughing, with vomiting of mucus, blue face and lips. Marcy and Hunt say: "It's effects are best shown where there is great and permanent structural change in the stomach. Excessive vomiting with great exertions, and extremely oppressive anxiety; violent pain in the stomach; oppression of the stomach, colic, obstinate constipation; diarrhea." In the last stages of consumption where there is much trouble with diarrhea, night sweats and general debility.

Dr. Hirschel says; "Cuprum is indicated in *catarrhal* affections of children, with suffocative spells. In *whooping cough,* if the spells are preceded by anxiety and attended by convulsions, stiffening of the body, losing of breath, slow recovery of respiration, suffocating spells and vomiting of food. Between the attacks, rattling noises in the chest. Especially indicative are the spasmus glottitis, protrusion of eyes, cyanosis, redness of the face, and bleeding from the mouth, nose and ears. In nervous asthma, with cough or spasms of the respiratory muscles, abdominal breathing, cold perspiration, small pulse, convulsion during and vomiting after the attack."

Aggravations, day and night, by inhaling cold air and during north and east winds.

Relieved by swallowing cold water.

DIGITALIS PURPUREA (MOIST) — A very slow pulse of intermittent, never rapid, but excited by the least movement; anasarca and dropsy, in organic diseases of the heart. Exceedingly prostrated after coughing; cough after eating, with vomiting of food.

This remedy has a special action upon the vagi; it's functions are interfered with, the bronchial mucous membranes become loaded with mucus; and we have a moist, loose, rattling cough, with an abundance of mucous expectoration; cyanotic symptoms of the face and sensation of an excessive determination of blood to the lungs, which produces difficulty in breathing. Baehr says: "Digitalis is particularly adapted to galloping phthisis with intense hectic fever from the commencement; the patient complains of palpitations of the heart, coughs up blood frequently, has no appetite; the cough must not be dry; bowels constipated, and the pulse is exceedingly quick. Dig. is the most reliable remedy to moderate hectic fever, but the dose must not be too small, nor should it be exceedingly large, because large doses are apt to excite the patient."

I am in the habit now, of using nothing but the active principle, Digitaline in the third centesimal; it acts like magic.

Meyhoffer says : "Digitalis is one of our most valuable medicines in passive congestion of the lungs an chronic catarrh resulting from a weak, dilated heart; irregularity and intermission of the pulse, scanty secretion of urine and œdematous swelling, are it's characteristic symptoms."

Aggravation, from getting heated; in a warm room, and from eating.

> **DROSERA ROTUNDIFOLIA (DRY)** — Deep, hoarse cough, worse after midnight. Paroxysms of spasmodic cough, with retching and vomiting. Perspires immediately on waking from sleep; cough so rapid in succession as it scarcely permits respiration in intervals.

This remedy, through the vagus, especially affects the larynx, trachea and bronchi, and is adapted to spasmodic, dry, hoarse cough, worse after midnight. Dr. Hirschel says : "The cough comes in fits, with long intervals; during the intervals, it is short, not exhausting, and the patient considers them trifles in comparison with the tormemting cough.

The fits begin mild and, short, they increase during the course of the disease; the cough is unceasing, in quick succession, forces one to sit up, always begins with titillation and renewed inspiration, till finally, after a few minutes up to a quarter of an hour or more vomiting of some mucus (rarely of food) sets in, which finishes the paroxysm. The cough seems to come from the very depth of the abdomen, as it were, convulses the muscles of the chest and abdomen, which remain painful for a long time, and the patient feels greatly exhausted after the fit. The fits are frequently aggravated by lying down at night. They are plainly of a spastic character, depending on an irritation of the vagus, and attack the bronchi. We meet them in whooping cough, in bronchial catarrh, after bronchitis in senility, in connection with emphysema, bronchiectasis, we only use the low dilutions, second or third, every three or four hours. Paroxysms always remind us of Drosera. This remedy has been given to cats and rabbits by Dr. Currie, and the pleural surface of both lungs was studded with what the microscope decided to be a true tubercle. The large doses the doctor forced down the cats explains to me how he found tubercles, a great portion of the liquid passed directly into the lungs and by it's mechanical irritation produced what he supposed to be tubercles; clinical experience does not corroborate Drosera's power of producing tubercles, and all such experiments where the medicine enters the air passages through force must prove abortive.

Aggravations, in the evening, after lying down and especially after midnight.

DULCAMARA (DRY) — Cough, from damp, cold atmosphere or from getting wet.

This remedy in my hands has never given any satisfaction

and I have finally ceased to use it, but other physicians claim to have good results from it, Hughes says : "They have to cough a long time to expel phlegm, especially in infants and old people, from threatened paralysis in the vagi." A catarrhal cough brought on by cold, damp weather. This remedy ought to be one of the first to choose, judging from the experience of physicians of high standing in the profession.

> **FERRUM METALLICUM (DRY)** — The least emotion, or exertion produces a red flushed face. Face becomes suddenly fiery red, with vertigo, ringing in the ears, palpitations of the heart and dyspnea; anæmia, with great paleness of the mucous membranes, especially that of the mouth; muscles feeble, easily exhausted from slight exertion. Loud bellows-sound of the heart from anæmia. Lienteria, stools of undigested food without pain; edematous swelling of the body, constant chilliness; evening fever similar to hectic. Hæmorrhagic tendency. Diseases, coincident with dropsical conditions, coldness of the whole body, especially nights.

This element in the constitution of our tissues acts in the two fold character of pabulum and medicine. In the present state of science it is often impossible to determine the exact limit where the nutritive action ceases, and the medicinal begins. Strictly speaking, iron is not what we would call a true cough remedy but it is so valuable in peculiar states of the system that we class it amongst our most valuable remedies. Dr. Rueckert has given us an admirable picture of it's indications. He says:

"1. Relaxation and weakness of the entire musculature and emaciation, weakness of digestion, coldness of the extremities.

2. Anæmia under the mast of plethora and congestion, accompanied by a whitish colour of the mucous membranes.

3. Pulmonary tuberculosis, especially in young florid subjects with a remarkable erethism of the vascular system, inclination to congestion towards the chest. But we will remind here of the property of Iron, in larger doses, to occasion hæmorrhages, a reason for which allopathic physicians do not give it in tuberculosis with an inclination to hæmorrhage.
4. Aphonia, very distressing.
5. Chronic, watery diarrhea in children, usually soon after eating and drinking, *without pain and effort,* mostly containing undigested substances."

"*Iron* is also indicated after previous abuse of *Iodine* (like wise after Arsenic and China), and what scrofulous patients have not already been over fed by *Iodine* (or a compound thereof) when they are transferred to us from allopaths."

Dr. Meyhoffer says : "*Iron* (acetate or perchloride)—Dry cough, from vascular congestion, with difficult and oppressed breathing, diminished or rough vesicular murmur and fine sibilant ronchi, spitting of blood or bronchial hæmorrhage. Small weak pulse; palpitations of the heart on the least muscular exertion, deficient gastric secretion; the food lies heavy on the stomach; bowels relaxed and discharging undigested food; suppressed menstruation or profuse flooding."

The cough of iron is predominantly dry, but in the morning the expectoration may be copious, either mucoid or purulent with oppressed, short breathing, worse in cold air and better in warm air.

Dr. Pope says: "The cases in which *Ferrum is* especially valuable are those in which the patient is usually between twenty and thirty years of age; family history is free from any hereditary taint or tubercle; he is of a sanguine temperament, of a florid complexion, with an active circulation and an easily excited nervous system; the disease has been excited by neglected catarrh, causes which originated malnutrition with frequent inflammatory attacks upon the pulmonary organs; epistaxis, hæmoptysis, headache, congestions in various parts, easily excited; hectic fever runs high, and the loss of strength is very rapid, there is dyspnea, vomiting of food or lienteria. For this form of phthisis Dr. C. Müller very confidently recommends the Perchloride of Ferrum, in doses of one to three drops, of the first to the sixth decimal dilution. Marcy and Hunt prefer the Pyrophosphate in the third trituration; this latter is my preference also.

In conclusion, we would add the practical remarks of Dr. C. Müller : "Cough, dry at night in bed, loose and more frequent when walking; chest painful above and behind the sternum, with burning after cough. The cough is appeased by eating. The night cough is most oppressive, and sometimes attended with spitting of blood; at other times, this occurs on rising in the morning. Tobacco and brandy cause aggravations, or increase the muco-purulent expectoration; dryness in the chest, but transiently relieved by drinking, with copious secretion of mucus. Shooting pains, and a sense of tightness between the shoulders, impeding movements of the joints. Shooting and tearing in the shoulder joints, the chest feels full and tight, with sanguine congestion; painful oppression which obliges one to be seated, and sometimes, amounts to a constrictive spasm; the respiration is noisy, as in sleep; the breathing, slow and painful, is ameliorated by walking, or by speaking, and when most preoccupied in reading or writing; it is most troublesome in bed and in the evening; *the pains are worse after eating,* I cannot characterize the sphere of iron better in phthisis, than in affirming it's indication by those very states in which allopaths have found counter indications and dangers. It is most suited for young and florid subjects, presenting a transient erethism of circulation, with congestive tendencies towards the chest and head. The special symptoms are: agitation and heating, easily induced by corporal movements and moral emotions; and, as a consequence, palpitations, dyspnea, cough, sudden flushes of the cheeks, epistaxis, hæmoptysis, quick fatigue and nervous excitability. Iron rarely fails to help these subjects. It may also be useful in cases of hectic fever, colliquation, with real weakness and emaciation—thus either at the beginning or towards the end of the malady. In the first instance a complete cure is often obtainable, especially when phthisis is not hereditary and impressed upon a cachectic constitution, much is to be hoped from iron when the hereditary germ breaks out in the midst of an apparently florid health; and it is well known that these cases are not the least serious. The palliation effected by iron in the third period often suffices to banish for a time the varied phenomena of hectic fever, while the gastric forces recuperate under it."

> **GELSEMIUM SEMPERVIRENS (DRY)** — Dry, hard, spasmodic, nervous cough; complete nervous aphonia; nervous, hysterical women afflicted with spinal or uterine cough.

This is a grand remedy for nervous, hysterical women, with a dry nervous cough, and for nervous, hysterical aphonia no remedy has given me such good satisfaction. It's cough indications are not yet fully demonstrated, but it has a very useful sphere in strictly neurotic, reflex coughs, with great debility of the cerebro-spinal nervous system.

> **HEPAR SULPHURIS (MOIST)** — Great disposition to take cold; sweats day and night without relief, especially about the chest, with a sour smell; cannot bear to be uncovered; coughs when any part of the body is uncovered; suppuration inevitable; second stage of cough, after it has become loose; hoarse, rattling, croupy cough; laryngo-tracheal catarrh with much hoarseness; great sensitiveness to cold air; abuse of mercury.

After the first stages of a cough have passed, and we commence to have a loose, hoarse, rattling cough, no more useful remedy in the *materia medica* can be found. Dr. Hirschel says: "Hepar sulphuris suits those cases which are so far advanced by Acon., Bry., Brom., Merc., Iod., or Spongia, that they have passed into the stage of resolution.

It is our most important remedy where, in acute forms, this resolution has been prepared, or in moist coughs, resting on a catarrhal or organic base, in the upper as well as in the lower respiratory organs. In croup, as well as in pneumonia, it can only be indicated in the second stage. It suits tuberculosis far less than cheesy and chronic pneumonia. It may also be indicated in gastric and intestinal catarrhs or complications, or in sympathetic cough, or in such ones extending from inflammations of adjacent parts of the larynx or in the lower parts, mucous rales, are important indications for this remedy, acting on the plasticity of these processes."

Dr. Guernsey says: "Hepar sulphuris—Rattling, *choking* cough; it seems as if the patient would *choke* while coughing; in croup, *whooping cough,* or in *catarrh,* usually worse towards morning, and after eating."

Dr. Holcomb says: "When there is hoarseness and soreness of the chest, and a cough which is moderately moist and then dry again."

Marcy and Hunt say: "Hepar is an important specific for the following characteristic symptoms; anxious, hoarse and wheezing respiration, much aggravated on lying down; attacks of suffocation, which force the patient to throw the head back, in order to take a breath; dyspnea; dry and hollow cough; cough with expectoration of mucus; hoarseness of voice; exacerbation of fever in the after part of the day, succeeded by night sweats. In cases which seem to have been connected with suppression of salt-rheum, or other eruptive diseases, or metastasis of arthritic inflammations. The patient has an unhealthy skin which cracks or chaps and runs into suppuration or ulceration from slight injuries; is subject to pimples and blotches; sweats from the slightest exertion, and profusely at night; mentally irritable, impatient; has vertigo with pain in the head; falling of hair; erysipelatous eruptions of the face; feeling of something sticking, a rough scraping or stinging stitches in the throat; rawness of the fauces, swollen tonsils; expectoration mixed with blood. Putrid taste in the mouth, loathing of food; vomiting; waterbrash."

Dr. Meyhoffer says: "Hepar sulphuris 2d or 3d decimal, one grain morning and evening, will not be unworthy of reliance in the chronic catarrh of scrofulous children and adults, especially when the morbid process shows a tendency to invade the pulmonary vesicles. This is the moment when careful auscultation will enable the physician to nip the bud in the further progress of catarrhal pneumonia by appropriate means of which Hepar is one of the most efficient. This substance, is not of minor importance in bronchitis engendered by swelling of the bronchial glands. In such cases the remedy must be continued as long as the improvement progresses. In subacute catarrhal processes, Hepar corresponds to the stage characterized by the incipient collection of mucus in the air tubes. As this fluid at that period is composed essentially of mucous cells, and contains but a small proportion of pus corpuscles, it is thus rendered particularly glutinous and sticky. Hence the violent and suffocative paroxysm of coughing, is often attended by retching which precedes it's expulsion."

Dr. S. Nichol says: "The characteristic cough of Hepar is a dry, rough and hollow cough; or the cough may be dry and crowing, coming on in violent paroxysms. The expectoration is generally mucoid, though sometimes a bloody froth is raised, and occasionally small, hard, tuberculous masses. The respiration is hoarse, anxious and wheezing. It is aggravated by lying down. The dyspnea is very marked, with suffocative attacks which force the patient to throw the head back in order to take a breath. The voice is hoarse and croaking. The fever which exacerbates towards evening is followed by night sweats."

Dr. Baehr says: "A characteristic indication for Hepar is a dry, spasmodic, barking cough, with a wheezing sound over the whole thorax, without any real mucous rales; it is a steady cough, increasing to dreadful paroxysms at intervals, with danger of suffocation; it is excited by every attempt to draw a long breath, and only results in the expectoration of a yellowish, tenacious mucus."

Aggravations at night, from cold north-east winds, and from eating or drinking anything cold.

Relieved from warmth in general, warm air and in warm wet weather.

HYOSCYAMUS NIGER (DRY) — Cough from purely nervous irritation. While lying down constant cough, which ceases soon after rising up, violent paroxysms of spasmodic, exhausting cough; patient is compelled to sit up in bed; great nervous excitability. In women, loud laughter at the approach of menses; lascivious furor; without modesty, she wishes to uncover and expose herself; paralysis of the sphincter muscles; cerebral functions greatly perverted.

The starting point and center of action of Hyoscyamus is in the cerebrum, and the cough is purely neurotic. Dr. Hirschel says: "Hyoscyamus differs from Belladonna in it's purely anti-nervous nature without any relation to the vasomotory element. The nightly aggravation of a dry spasmodic, titillating cough in the trachea, aggravated by lying down, is most important. It has frequently disappointed me." So it has me, probably I have given it too high. Dr. Holcomb gives it in the pure tincture, one drop after every paroxysm of coughing, and says it is followed by magical relief.

Agrravations at night, especially when lying down; by cold air, and by eating and drinking.

Relieved by sitting up, and warm atmosphere.

> **IGNATIA AMARA (DRY)** — Diseases brought on from deep grief, with much sighing and sobbing; cannot sleep from deep, suppressed grief, entirely absorbed in grief; faint, all gone feeling in the pit of the stomach (solar plexus); hysterical element predominates; excessive flatulence; convulsive twitching; symptoms change often from joy to sadness; dry, hard spasmodic cough (globus hystericus).

Cough in patients who are suffering from suppressed grief, where there is not much organic disease of the air passages. They may be termed as hysterical, spinal reflux cough, always dry in nature. Ignatia will be of much service. Dr. Hirschel strikes the true key for it's use when he says: "Ignatia is only suitable for coughs of central origin, as from spinal irritation (hysteria), or where hysterical persons, catarrhal, laryngeal and tracheal affections take on a nervous character. Perhaps, also, in bronchial asthma, and angina pectoris of such patients; the cough is tickling, dry, as from dust or sulphur vapours, constriction in the pit of the throat, with globus hystericus and similar symptoms." Dr. Guernsey says: "Ignatia has a very troublesome cough, usually dry, arising from some irritation in the pit of the stomach.

Aggravations : Like Nux, the symptoms are aggravated by contact, motion, open air, mental affections, anger and grief.

Relieved by changing position and in warm air.

> **IODIUM (DRY)** — Remarkable sense of weakness and loss of breath on going up stairs; low cachectic, scrofulous people; in women, great emaciation of the mammæ, with copious menstruation, or long lasting uterine hæmorrhages; enlarged glands, especially the thyroid. Dry cough predominates. Dark hair and eyes.

The physiologico-pathological centre for the action of Iod. is upon the glandular system. Small doses increase their secretions and sometimes intense salivation has followed it's exhibition. Atrophy of the mammæ and testes are prominent symptoms of Iod. It's specific action upon the thyroid gland and upper portion of the air passages, are very marked and prominent, and of great practical utility. Dr. Hirschel says that "*Iodine, Bromine* and *Spongia* have this in common; that they especially cure the affections of the upper parts of the respiratory organs; that they correspond to dry cough, if of catarrhal, inflammatory or organic origin. All are deeply penetrating and reliable remedies. *Spongia* might be considered the most volatile and dynamic; *Bromium* is materially incisive, forcible and helps quickly; *Iod.* is the strongest, but most slow in action. They are the chief remedies in the affections of the larynx and trachea (catarrhs, inflammations, especially croup, changes in texture); also in stenosis of the glottis. *Iod.* alone has also some relations to the bronchi, and even to the pulmonary tissue. According to the symptoms we find in *Bromium* dry, croupy cough with scraping titillation and hoarseness; the latter is a special indication for *Bromium*. Where small follicles are found on the posterior mucous membrane of the pharynx, extending from there to the larynx and producing a continuous titillating cough, *Bromium* is specific; also in swelling of the mucous membrane of the fauces and pharynx. The larynx is painful to the touch. In *Iodine,* the cough is also dry, croupy, with the well known sound and titillation; sensation of soreness in the larynx, barking with gray or white, salty, sweetish expectoration; shrill whistling and rattling in the chest, sawing, hissing respiration and oppression. The subjective sensation of soreness and pain frequently extends to the upper third of the sternum. Hoarseness, difficult speech, expectoration of tough mucus. I have frequently witnessed from *Iod.* splendid effects in long standing laryngeal catarrhs with the above symptoms. It alleviates in tuberculosis; in croup it the is last anchor where *Spongia* and *Bromium* fail. It is not easy to select from these three remedies; each may be indicated according to the circumstances. *The more plastic the exudation, the more Iod. is indicated.*

Anatomically, we might say *Spongia* is more suitable for stasis, simple inflammation; *Bromium* for swelling and hypertrophy of the mucous membranes; *Iod.* for the exudation. *Spongia*, whose indications generally correspond to those of Iod. (whistling, short, dry, barking cough at night and also during the day time, with a painful sensation in the larynx), is, in the main, the most important remedy at the outset of croup; frequently cuts it short, and acts specifically and in the shortest time in pseudo-croup, or in the closely related inflammatory or highly catarrhal forms; also in influenza. On account of it's volatile action, it suits far less the organic and chronic forms of cough than the related *Bromium* and *Iod.*

Dr. Meyhoffer says: "An effort to give precise clinical indications for Iod. seems like a difficult one, as the horizon of it's curative action appears its with the progress of therapeutical knowledge. Though the pathogenetic phenomena of this metalloid are most extensive, they give *a priori*, in numerous instances, no clue to the vitalizing manifestations it operates in disease. For example, as regards the respiratory surface, we meet within the range of it's salutary influence the dry, congestive catarrh, profuse bronchorrhea and catarrhal pneumonia, with all the intermediary morbid conditions. Still one link exists which binds all these so contradictory symptoms together, and this is *irritation.* Torpidity and atony of the ventilating apparatus does not lie within it's range."

"Iod. has, in common with Cod liver oil, the property of being exquisitely adapted to delicate constitutions, with a quick pulse, tendency to bronchial and pulmonary congestion and hæmorrhage. For the same reason it is also an excellent remedy for over grown lads, with a weak chest and dry cough, subject to spitting blood and cardiac palpitations. The cough which this substance relieves is always more or less severe, the expectoration may be scanty or copious; fine or coarse rattles and sibilant ronchi give way to it's influence. Swelling of the cervical and bronchial glands, nocturnal sweats, great weakness and progressive emaciation, not withstanding a good appetite and regular functions of the bowels are important confirmative indications for the exhibition of Iod. We use it in the third and higher dilutions; the Iod. of Potassium from the first to the third. The latter appears to act better when the affection of the air tubes is connected with or complicated by rheumatism."

Dr. Baehr says: "Iod. is undoubtedly one of our most important remedies in confirmed phthisis; it only suits, however, after the expectoration has become purulent. This remedy effects more frequently then any other, curative results, provided we do not obstinately insist upon giving only small doses. Iodine 6× sometimes has a good effect, but Iodine 1× is often indispensable; nor need any unpleasant effects be apprehended from the use of such large doses. Iodine is more particularly indicated if tuberculosis is the result of scrofulosis, in the case of young and robust individuals; if diarrhea is present, Iod. does not act favorably as a rule."

"Chronic catarrh of scrofulous and mercurialized individuals, or remaining after croup or other acute affections, or complicated with chronic pharyngeal catarrh, are affections lying within the range of Iod. The most prominent symptomatic indications are the following : disposition to take cold, and a long duration of the acute stage; the larynx is painful when pressed upon; burning, sore pains in the larynx confined to a definite spot, felt especially during cough; embarrassed respiration; wheezing inspirations, causing real attacks of dyspnea, especially at night; a good deal of hawking, with difficulty in bringing up tenacious mucus; a high degree of hoarseness, even aphonia; tickling in the larynx frequently causing paroxysms of cough without expectoration, or else with scanty expectoration of a tenacious mucus, sometimes mixed with streaks of blood. The general organism is very much affected by the disease. The presence of ulcers points more particularly to Iod.

Aggravations at night, by warm air and warmth in general; going up stairs, lying in bed and lying on the painful side. Relieved by cold air, or a cool place and after eating.

IPECACUANHA (MOIST) — Constant nausea; constant but unavailable desire to vomit; vomiting gives no relief, the nausea still remains; severe suffocative cough; asthmatic cough, second stage of catarrh, when the cough begins to be loose. The chest seems full of phlegm, but does not yield to coughing.

The Ipecac cough does not have an organic base, but is of a simple catarrhal origin mixed up with the neurotic element; loose, spasmodic cough, with constriction of the air passages, and a large accumulation of mucus in them. Dr. Hirschel says: "Catarrhal, or spasmodic *titillating* cough, or *suffocating cough* with dyspnea, nausea, vomiturition, especially at the end of a paroxysm, or with expectoration of a scanty, albuminous, *nauseous* mucus; *or if* mucous rales and vomiting of food (but in a less degree than from Tartar emetic), are present. The inclination to vomit, the absence of any inflammatory irritation and the tendency to resolution, are indications for this remedy. Gastric catarrh, bronchial asthma, more in bronchial than in laryngeal affections. In whooping cough only towards the end. It has special relations to the vagus, and suits women and children well." Dr. S. Nichol, while treating bronchitis, says: "Ipecac. is one of the principal remedies for the bronchial catarrhs of infancy and childhood in it's action, closely resembling Tartar emetic. It is almost indispensable in these peculiar attacks, partly neurosis, partly phlogosis—a kind of mixture of asthma and bronchitis—which frequently occurs in young children, and which are so fatal when treated by our medical step brethren. It is indicated by loud and sonorous mucous rales in the chest, and wheezing respiration. There is great dyspnea coming on in paroxysms in the evening, continuing with slight remissions during the night, and intermitting distinctly through the day. The cough is convulsive, suffocative, and relief from this partial suffocation is had when vomiting takes place. During the vomiting the face assumes a bluish hue, and bleeding from the nostrils may take place. A slight degree of spasm in the glottis is not unfrequent and there may be convulsive twitchings or even spasmodic rigidity of the child's body. Sometimes inspite of the mucous rales, the cough is dry; though, as Baehr remarks, this is certainly not according to it's physiological symptoms. As to the dose, Dr. Meyhoffer remarks that a low dilution is essential in obtaining prompt relief, and Baehr remarks that, at any rate, we know from experience that a smaller dose than a grain of the second trituration does not produce a reliable effect." I have used the remedy extensively and have had excellent results from the twelfth decimal trituration of the root which is a very different thing from the twelfth dilution of the tincture.

Baehr says : "If the cough had lasted for some time and been neglected, the indications for Ipecac are tolerably precise and unmistakable. If, instead of the usual tenacious and scanty mucus, a large quantity of simple catarrhal mucus accumulates, so that cough is preceded and accompanied by loud rales; if every paroxysm of cough is attended with vomiting, not at the end, but at the commencement; if a paroxysm is excited by the ingestion of every trifling quantity of food of drink, Ipecac deserves a preference over every other remedy."

Aggravations at night, also in the morning, by exertion; in the warm air of a room and on stepping into the open air.

KALIUM BICHROMICUM (MOIST) — Cough with expectoration of tough, stringy mucus; inflammation of the pharynx and fauces, parts smooth and red; adapted to the second stage, especially in tedious cases, where the mucus appears to be loose, but it sticks to the parts very tenaciously, and can be drawn out in long strings; chronic catarrh of the nose and fauces; light hair and eyes.

For sub-acute and chronic tedious cases of cough, where the large bronchi, trachea, larynx and fauces are involved; where the cough seems to be loose, and what is expectorated is very sticky and ropy. Dr. Meyhoffer says : "Inhalations and the internal use of *Kali bi.* form our standard course of treatment in those numerous cases of common bronchitis vacillating between the acute and the torpid inveterate character of the disease. A certain degree of irritation, vascular congestion and moderate muco-purulent expectoration marks the morbid state ready to give way to the specific working of this salt. Inhalations, however, do good service in bronchial dilatation with fetid breath and expectoration. The sputa soon undergo a favorable change of aspect, while they lose at the same time their offensive odor and diminish in quantity. If the catarrh be attended by periosteal or rheumatic pains of a chronic character, all hesitation as to the selection of this medicine must subside."

Dr. Hirschel says : "Kali bi., with it's dry, titillating cough, expelled at short intervals, and ulcerative pain in the larynx, is related to Bromine, Spongia and Iod., but suits medium and tedious cases better. It's characteristic symptom is a *smooth or follicular inflammatory redness of the pharynx and fauces.*"

Dr. Lilienthal says, speaking of croup : "Suits fat, chubby children; onset is gradual and insidious; constant hoarse voice; cough at intervals, hoarse, dry, barking, metallic; deglutition painful; tonsils and larynx red, swollen; covered with a false membrane, difficult to detach, with expectoration of tough, stringy mucus."

Dr. Nichol says : "Where the sputa is difficult and tenacious, and comes up in long strings of opaque white mucus, the preference should be given to *Kali bi.* This indication of Kali has been verified over and over again, and we owe it to Dr. Drysdale."

Baehr remarks : "Very seldom, however, a favorable effect will be witnessed in cases where emphysema has already set in, for this reason the remedy is better adapted to chronic catarrhs of recent origin, that had taken the place of an acute disease, than to inveterate cases."

Dr. Guernsey says : "Kali bi.; cough, with expectoration of tough, stringy mucus; it sticks in the throat, causing a choking sensation, sticks to the tongue, teeth and lips, and in attempting to remove it from these parts, it will be drawn out into long strings."

Aggravations, after eating, on awaking and on inspiration.

KALIUM CARBONICUM (DRY) — Cough brought on from cold and damp weather; very violent, mostly dry cough, commencing at 3 A.M.; if mucus is dislodged it is not raised, but falls back in the stomach; severe stitching pain is the most characteristic symptom of this remedy; all the symptoms are regularly worse about 3 A.M.; swelling over the upper eyelid in the morning, looking like a little bag; chronic organic coughs; acts on the lower portion of right lung.

For old, very hard, chronic, dry, racking coughs, with stitching pains in the chest and back; worse in cold, damp weather, or brought on by cold and damp, and aggravated about 3 A.M., Kali c. is *the* remedy. Dr. Meyhoffer says: "Kali c., in a very low dilution, proves a useful auxiliary in those chronic forms of bronchitis which only fall under the physician's observation when cold and damp weather have induced vascular irritation. A severe, sometimes spasmodic cough, torments the patient day and night, and the effort to bring up a few lumps of grayish mucus often determines retching and vomiting. The breathing, usually easy, becomes difficult and labored after the frequent paroxysms of coughing. The general health of such persons is good, the nutrition nowise disturbed, and should they belong to the working class, they do not even leave off their employment during such attacks."

Dr. Rafka says: "Kali c. 6×, is indicated by a dry, titillating cough, with stinging in the larynx, pains in the chest, choking, violent headache, exhaustion after the attack, which commonly sets in at night, is also useful in titillating cough during menses, and in incipient tuberculosis."

Aggravations, at night, especially after midnight, on motion; by cold damp air, or becoming cold; while eating; from deep inspiration and from lying on the side. Relieved by warm, dry air.

> **KALIUM BROMATUM (MOIST)** — Not much cough, but great hypersecretion of muco-purulent matter, with dyspnea; great depression of nervous centres, with loss of memory and general lethargy; inertia of the genital organs; great atony of the larynx; confluent acne; nervous spasmodic cough; chronic and sub-acute cases.

Having never used this remedy for cough frequently enough to form a correct judgment upon it's merits, I will give the practical experience of others who have used it. Dr. Meyhoffer says the "Bromide of Potassium, somewhat resembles Iod. in it's action upon scrofulous diseases, differs, however, as much from it as sub-acute inflammation does from passive congestion. We have experienced the efficacy of the Bromide in that form of bronchial catarrh which is characterized by almost total absence of cough, with great hypersecretion of muco-purulent matter and dyspnea caused by muscular exertion. The diminished or suspended reflex motor action of the bronchial nerves belongs especially to the pathogenesis of Bromide of the Potassium, and unless the larynx is involved in the morbid process, this salt will rarely bring relief."

Dr. E. M. Hale, in speaking of croup, says: "But no remedy acts so promptly palliative in all cases, and curative in many, as *Kali br.* in spasmodic croup. The symptoms are at once arrested."

"Whooping cough—the spasmodic action disappeared in about five days, leaving a simple bronchial catarrh. It removes the anxiety and the vomiting; improves the appetite and increases the strength."—*Dr. Beaufort.*"

"*Nervous cough* during pregnancy—threatening abortion; the cough was dry, hard and almost incessant; Opium, Bell., etc., were tried for two months, without benefit. Bromide of Potash, 30 grains a day, cured in a few hours."—*Dr. Cerson.*

The spasmodic element seems to be a prominent symptom in the cough of *Kali br.*

> **KALI HYDRIODICUM**—Very fatiguing, dry, hard cough; walking or going up stairs causes great shortness of breath; syphilitic subjects with glandular swellings; mercurial or syphilitic rheumatism; syphilitic, aphthous sore mouth; phthisis with expectoration of *green mucus;* rheumatic pains in the limbs, worse nights; very sensitive to the least cold air; old syphilitic subjects; syphilitic or scrofulous skin diseases; asthma.

The action of this remedy is very similar to Iod., especially in scrofulous swellings of glands and goitre, but differs in many points. Oppressive, dry, painful cough, frequently accompanied with asthma, is the great sphere for the use of Iodide of Potash. Dr. Meyhoffer says : "The lower dilutions, 1st and 2nd, from four to eight drops daily, form one of our standard prescriptions, whenever no special symptoms indicate the use of another drug. In glandular swellings it cannot be omitted. Dry, irritating cough, with scanty and rather frothy than mucoid expectoration, or none at all; obstinate tickling and irritation in the trachea; prolonged expiration with sensation of tightness in the chest and shortness of breath are the leading symptoms for the selection of this remedy."

Dr. W. H. Hitchman says : "Kali i. is beneficial, indeed, often of great service in those cases where there exists a considerable degree of irritation in the bronchial tubes, especially the larger channels, with a hollow dry cough, day and night, but worse towards evening; or cough with scanty, viscid, ropy expectoration; heat in the chest; burning, tickling irritation in the larynx; quick, anxious, laborious respiration, with hoarseness; slight abdominal pains, often scarcely noticeable, but at the same time most insidious, dangerous and fatal in their ultimate results. They are augmented by pressure; fullness and tension of the belly, particularly a *deep seated tightness,* as if the integument and muscles glided over the too tightly stretched and thickened peritoneum or serous membrane; coughing and deep breathing are painful, and there is feverishness with emaciation."

Dr. Baehr says: "If the influenza left the patient with a troublesome cough and a gray, sweetish-salt expectoration; wheezing and rattling in the chest, *Kali i.* proved an admirable remedy. This remedy is likewise excellent for the remaining hoarseness or even aphonia, but should not be given in too small doses." Patient is very apt to have chronic nasal catarrh, excited and aggravated by cold; severe bone pains, where the bones are swollen; violent headache with hard a lupus.

Most symptoms appear during rest, especially in cold damp weather and are relieved by motion. Rheumatic pains are much better during motion.

> **KREOSOTUM (MOIST)** — Putrid diseases, with great acridity of the secretions, livid complexion, disposition sad and irritable. Oedema and fetid sweat of the feet; paroxysmal moist cough, the lungs seem loaded with mucus, but cannot expectorate without long and continued coughing. In women the menses are too frequent, too profuse and last too long.

In organic affections of the mucous membranes of the bronchi, this is a remedy of great value. It's symptoms are very similar to those of Pulsatilla, the distinction being this: the cases that are adapted to Kreosotum are more deeply seated, have lasted longer, and if in the case of a woman, the menses are too often, too profuse and last too long, whereas in Pulsatilla, the menses are apt to be delayed and are too scanty. Kreos. is adapted to coughs that have passed from the dry, first stage, and the second stage has fully set in; the cough sounds very loose, the upper bronchi is loaded with mucus, but expectoration is very difficult. The cough has much of the nervous element about it, which makes it paroxysmal in character. Marcy and Hunt say of Kreos. "Constant, spasmodic, violent cough, accompanied by violent retching; the expectoration is copious, mucoid and purulent; the patient cannot lie down without great distress; stitching pain in the chest; bitter taste in the mouth; cadaverous breath; frequent greenish, watery diarrhea; hectic fever; copious secretion of the mucous membranes and abscesses which are excessively offensive in character, accompanied with depression of nervous power. In these conditions, says Dr. Kurtz, Kreos. is much more effectual than Arsenicum, which is usually prescribed—('Hygeia.')"

Cough with pain in the chest and sternum compelling one to press the hand on it; great sleepiness and profound sleep; frequent desire to take a deep breath on account of a sensation of heavings on the chest.

Shortness of breath, with sensation of heaviness on the chest; stitches in the chest, above and in the region of the heart, with oppression of breathing on the right side, extending under the shoulder blade, arresting breathing.

The chest feels bruised, especially in the sternum.*

Aggravation in the open air; morning and evening ; by motion and from eating cold food.

LACHESIS MUTUS (DRY) — Very unhappy and distressed after sleep; throat exceedingly sensitive, cannot bear the least touch of a finger; she cannot bear any pressure, not even of the clothes, upon the uterine region. Hot flushes at climacteric, with frequent fainting spells.

---

* "Dull pain under the sternum every morning when turning over in bed; hyperesthesia of bronchial mucous membrane during bad weather, with occasional bloody sputa. The 30× cured."—DR. REYNOLDS.

> When anything touches the larynx the latter is not only sensitive, but it feels as though it would suffocate him; touching the throat causes a dry hacking cough; dry spasmodic cough, worse nights, with a choking sensation in the throat; greatly aggravated by sleep; empty swallowing is perfectly agonizing.

This remedy is more suitable to a neurotic, reflex-spasmodic cough, than to those with an organic base.

Dr. Guernsey says : "Cough excited by pressing, even lightly upon the larynx; clothing must be removed from about the part—it's pressure excites the cough. Cough as soon as one *falls into a sound sleep, often with choking, as if suffocation was inevitable.* In croup, cough excited by a sensation, as if a crumb of bread were sticking in the throat, or some other substance, with frequent hawking and swallowing."

Dr. Holcomb says : "Lachesis acts beautifully for tickling, worrying night cough with a sensation of a lump in the throat, sensitiveness of the larynx, especially when after a long, dry paroxysm, there is suddenly a profuse expectoration of frothy mucus."

Dr. Meyhoffer says; "Lachesis and Naja, always contribute to allay the harassing cough, secondary either to nervous palpitations or organic alterations of the heart. Deficient nervous influence of the par vagum, dilatation and fatty degeneration of the heart, constitute the sphere in which these poisons display their restorative influence. The contingent symptoms of one or the other of these remedies. They are valuable auxiliaries of Arsenic, Phosphorus and Digitalis, and when properly employed, contribute largely to maintain the equilibrium between the function of the heart and the capillary circulation."

Aggravations after every sleep; at night; touching the throat or larynx; damp cold weather and from acids.

> **LYCOPODIUM CLAVATUM (MOIST)** —Excessive accumulation of flatulence in the stomach and bowels; constant sensation of satiety; the least morsel of food causes a a sensation of fullness up to the throat; much borborygmus, especially in the left hypochondrium; constant sense of fermentation in the abdomen, like a pot of yeast working; obstinate constipation; great excess of lithic acid gravel in the urine, so much that the urine seems filled with it; cold clammy, night sweats; great disposition to take cold at every change of the weather; loose rattling cough, with great difficulty in breathing during the paroxysm of cough; perspiration only on the chest and head, with great debility in diseases of the lungs. Fan like motion of the alæ nasi.

This is a grand remedy for cough and greatly resembles Pulsatilla, Hepar sulphuris and Kreosotum. The cough is loose, but remains in the lungs very tenaciously. The sputa is thick, yellow or greenish. Dr. Meyhoffer says: "A long time was necessary to conquer my repugnance to the use of Lycopodium, excited by the exaggerated laudations of it's medicinal virtues which I had been condemned to listen to; now I have, on the contrary, to guard against falling into the same error myself. The fact is, since I learned to appreciate it's efficacy in chronic pneumonia, I have not failed to observe also it's vitalizing influence in those forms of bronchitis characterized by copious muco-serous, or mucopurulent secretion. These morbid phenomena being habitually the result of more or less serious alterations, it follows that Lycopodium acts favorably in dilatation of the air tubes and senile catarrh. Constant tickling cough, worse at night, numerous loud mucous rattles, with rare and scanty sputa, are symptoms lying especially within the range of it's action. But the varieties of bronchitis above mentioned are often attended or complicated by the phenomena of abdominal vascular obstruction and atony of the alimentary canal or by those of the acid diathesis. The signs which arise in such circumstances, as congestion of the liver, flatulency, obstinate constipation, cachectic complexion, red gravel in the urine and acid dyspepsia, are all within the range of the influence of Lycopodium. Low dilutions of it are not ineffectual, but higher ones work better."

Baehr says: "Lycopodium is suitable for old people, if emphysema and marked changes in the bronchial mucous membrane have taken place; there is constant tickling in the throat, loud rales with scanty or unfrequent expectoration of a gray colour and saltish taste, nightly exacerbations. Usually Lycopodium is indicated in moist mucous, or muco-purulent coughs, but Dr. C. Wesselhoeft has had fine results with it in dry cough, day and night; in feeble, emaciated patients, the cough being worse nights.

Dr. Hitchman says: "Lycopodium will almost invariably afford signal relief when there is fluent coryza, with cough and hoarseness; stuffing of the nostrils; formication or an ant like crawling in the windpipe at night; dry cough in the morning; cough after drinking; cough which affects the chest; a loose cough with spitting of purulent matter, like confirmed consumption; short breathing in children; constant oppression with suffocation on doing the least work; painful stitches in the left part of the chest, with a bruised feeling; beating of the heart in bed; herpetic spots on the neck and chest; pain in the loins in bed; stitches in the back after stooping; dragging in the shoulder blades; stiffness of the nape of the neck; boring pains in the arms; twitching in the arms during sleep; dry skin; the patient complains of having lost all strength in the arms and having cold feet; moreover when the cough is troublesome, materially worse at night and attended with thirst, quickness of pulse, subsequent tendency to moist skin, expectoration grayish, saltish or yellowish, with oppression about the bronchial tubes, this medicine is strikingly indicated."

Dr. Pope says: "Few medicines are so valuable in pulmonary phthisis as this, when persistently used. The cough, gastric irritation, exhaustion and intercurrent attacks of pleurisy, are wonderfully mitigated by it."

"Expectoration of large quantities of pus; cough day and night; hectic fever; circumscribed redness of the cheeks; great emaciation of the upper part of the body, while the lower portion is enormously distended."—*Raue.*

Dr. Goullon says: "Lycopodium is closely related to Sulphur, which is also contained in the plant from which we obtain the Lycopodium seeds. For this reason alone the second designation of Lycopodium, *sulphur vegetabilis*, is justified. Loose cough during the day, hoarseness and paroxysms of suffocation are present at night, as a general thing, if suffocative paroxysms interchange with free intervals."

"Where the right side is more affected, the cough loose, full and deep, *sounding as though the entire parenchyma were softened, the patient raising a whole mouthful of mucus at a time, which in colour is a light rust, not much unlike that of Bryonia, but not so thick, more stringy and easily separated,* and if, in addition, there should be present a "fan like" motion of the alæ nasi of the nose. Lycopodium 200, will almost certainly afford relief within twelve hours."—*C. Pearson, M.D.*

In prescribing Lycopodium it's action on the digestive canal and liver should never be lost sight of. The dyspeptic symptoms, such as *flatulence* and *constipation*, are nearly always one of the most prominent indications for this remedy.

"Lycopodium is a most effective remedy in obstinate cough, aggravated at night, with constant tickling in the throat, shown by the restlessness of the little patient, with constant handling of the front of the neck—loud rales with scanty expectoration, of tough salty mucus and grayish colour. The respiration of Lycopodium is predominant with the moist sound, while the respiration of Pulsatilla, Sepia and Silicea are marked by the predominance of the dry sound."—*T. Nichol, M.D.*

Aggravations, evenings from four to eight o'clock, and again at midnight; from exertion, lying down, from cold drinks, from deep inspiration and from high winds. Relieved, usually, in a warm atmosphere and by warm food.

> **MERCURIUS SOLUBILIS (DRY)** — Symptoms greatly aggravated at night, and in cold, damp weather. Spongy gums that bleed easily; salivation; thick yellow coated tongue, with very fetid breath, aphthæ of the mouth and fauces; enlarged glands, especially those of the mouth. Much perspiration, that does not relieve; jaundice; muco-sanguinolent stools, or serous diarrhea; high coloured urine; hectic fever. Dry cough, with roughness and burning down to the sternum, showing that the mucous membrane is inflamed; ropy sputum.

This remedy is adapted to a dry cough, that is passing into a moist cough, after the primary symptoms have been nearly subdued by Acon., Bell., or Bry., and is greatly aggravated at night. It chronic bronchitis, Mercury is also of great value where there is a copious secretion of mucus, or muco-purulent expectoration with exhaustive night sweats, &c.

Dr. Hirschel says: "How the allopaths, and more still their patients, are to be pitied, that their school should lack a knowledge of *Mercurius* (sol.), as a cough remedy. Where is there a more certain, a more specifically acting remedy for the appropriate kinds of cough of a catarrhal, inflammatory, organic nature, running from the fauces through the trachea and down to the finest bronchi, decisive in acute affections, ameliorating in the chronic, slime-loosening resolvent, restorative! Where *roughness, burning, feeling of soreness* from the fauces down to the sternum, hoarseness of voice, dry cough, raw, concussive, exhaustive, naturally exacerbated; sputum ropy, watery, spittle like, nasty bloody; catarrhal headache, coryza, diarrhea, fever, non-ameliorating night sweats—here is the real province of *Mercurius*. It's place is some where after Acon., before Bry., or Puls., or Hep., or Tartar emetic; also ushering in the turning point, critically intervening, so that the last mentioned may finish the affair. *Mercurius* is the sovereign remedy for bronchitis, and of inflammatory bronchial catarrh."

Dr. T. Nichol, speaking of capillary bronchitis, says: "Merc. is an excellent remedy for this form of bronchitis. The cough is dry, racking and violent, especially in the evening and until midnight. It is excited by tickling, or a sensation of dryness in the chest, with expectoration of yellowish, tenacious mucus, sometimes tinged with blood. Each paroxysm of cough is preceded by anxious oppression, with hoarseness and coryza; violent fever, with a disposition to perspire, without any relief from it; the tongue is thickly coated, and the alternate chills and heat are succeeded by exhausting sweats. This remedy acts best in repeated doses of the fourth and fifth trituration, dry on the tongue." In chronic bronchitis, "paroxysms of cough at night, with coldness during the paroxysms and distress for breath; there is a good deal of sweetish or saltish mucus and blood; soreness and ulcerative pain in the air passages, especially during the cough, and the cough may give rise to nausea and actual vomiting."

One of the most prominent indications for this remedy is a constant alternation of chills and fever; the fever is often very high, with a remarkable sensitiveness to the most trifling changes of temperature; thick, yellow coated tongue and diarrhea, with great longing for icy cold drinks, although they aggravate the cough.

In pneumonia Dr. Müller says: "The hepatization of a portion of lung continues, and the critical sputa is entirely wanting; the cough is dry, not frequent, very rough and fatiguing, with violent irritation and urging to cough; the dyspnea remains unaltered, the fever is continuous and lentescent, with profuse and exhausting sweats; the urine is scanty and dim, the colour of the skin is sallow, grayish, the patient is troubled with gastro-intestinal catarrh. Under these circumstances, Mercury is indicated so much more if the disease is seated in a scrofulous or dyscrasic organism."

Dr. Baehr says: "The selection of Mercury in broncho-pneumonia may be justified by it's admirable action in bronchitis; for it cannot be denied that the greatest danger proceeds from this quarter, and that, after the removal of the bronchial symptoms, the remaining pneumonia is comparatively insignificant. A third form of pneumonia, which is particularly adapted to *Mercurius,* is the catarrhal form or lobular pneumonia, which has an entirely different meaning from the former. As soon as we have reason, in a case of bronchitis, whooping cough, etc., to suspect the formation of a small foci of exudation, Mercurius will first commend itself to our judgment as a remedial agent, and we shall have before our eyes an image of epidemic influenza. In tubercular pneumonia we have never noticed any good effects from Mercurius.

"In phthisis caused by syphilis, Hartmann says: "I have cured several cases of it perfectly. I commenced the treatment with several doses of *Merc.,* when syphilitic ulcers were still visible in the throat, extending deep down, involving the larynx, occasioning hoarseness and that ominous cough with irritation, together with the burning and tickling in the region of the larynx. If large doses of *Merc.* had already been taken, I gave Merc. cor., after which the ulcers soon disappeared, and the affection of the larynx became much less. There were cases where this success did not occur; I then employed with a similar benefit the *red precipitate*. If the patient had been poisoned with large doses of Mercury, I gave *Nit. ac.*"

Aggravations, at night; from getting warm in bed; from rapid motion; lying down on the right side and cold, damp air.

> **MERCURIUS PROTO-IODATUS (MOIST)** — Secondary syphilis; scrofulous subjects, with chronic nasal or pharyngeal catarrh; enlarged and indurated glands, especially the parotid and inguinal glands; buccal, submaxillary and tonsils greatly enlarged, inflamed and very painful, with a constant flow of tough, ropy mucus; mucous membranes raw, the epithelium being entirely destroyed; complete destruction of the respiratory mucous membrane, with loose, rattling cough, and copious mucoid or mucopurulent expectoration.

This is one of the most valuable remedies in the *materia medica* in loose, rattling cough, where the bronchi are loaded with mucus, or a muco-purulent matter, the bronchial mucous membrane seems to be undergoing complete solution on account of the great secretion of mucus. This kind of a cough is apt to be engrafted upon a scrofulous subject that has long been suffering with chronic catarrh. The mucous membrane of the pharynx and nose is greatly congested and swollen, that of the nose so much that in many cases it is impossible to breathe through it; fetid breath, &c.

Dr. Meyhoffer says : "*Iodide of Mercury* corresponds more particularly to subacute processes arising from the influence of cold or atmospheric variations; protracted cases, after *Bell.*, when the parts are much swollen, dark coloured, with much hawking, coughing, and viscid muco-purulent expectoration, particularly in the morning. In follicular laryngitis, *Iodide of Mercury* has been highly commended in the more acute forms, from the first to the third trituration; but although the more acute symptoms have yielded rapidly to it's influence, we never attained, by means of this salt alone, perfect absorption of the swollen follicles."

In a chronic tubercular sore throat and laryngitis, the fauces and epiglottis have a deep livid, purplish hue, and the secretions are thin and acrid, and frequently ptyalism, with very fetid breath. There is apt to be chronic nasal catarrh, with a vast amount of mucus in the nose, much of which descends through the posterior nares into the throat. In membranous croup, the pseudo-membrane is not only in the bronchi, trachea and larynx, but is located upon the tonsils, uvula, velum palati and pharynx, not fibrinous, but of feeble organization. Where the membrane is tough, Kali bi., Iod. or Sanguinaria are more appropriate. The cough is very loose and expectoration quite easy. Much languor and prostration; bowels inclined to be loose; dark red urine, and tongue coated thickly yellow. Especially if the patient has had syphilis and is suffering from it's secondary effects.

Aggravation in a warm room, at night during rest, and early in the morning.

Relieved in cool air and by active exercise.

NITRICUM ACIDUM (DRY) — Chronic cough, engrafted upon subjects with some virulent poison in their system, such as syphilitic, mercurial or scrofula. Especially cachectic, broken down people, suffering from secondary syphilis, with caries of the bones, emaciation and great debility. Spreading ulcers in the mouth and throat; fetid breath, parotid and submaxillary glands swollen; bloody saliva; complete aphonia; mouth full of fetid ulcers, affecting the fauces and nares; chronic looseness of the bowels; urine smells like that of horses, extremely offensive; takes cold very easily; sensation as if a sharp splinter was being stuck into the affected part; colliquative night sweats that are very offensive; great emaciation; constipation.

In the last stages of consumption, Nit. ac. may be indicated when there is a loose cough, but as a rule, the cough is inclined to be dry when this remedy is called for. Dr. Hirschel says: "Nit. ac. has it's sphere of action in chronic inflammatory forms of cough, in ulcerous or tuberculous processes of the larynx and bronchi; in pneumonia which tends towards phthisis; in cirrhosis of the lungs and especially in chronic catarrhs combined with angina pectoris or diseases of the heart."

Dr. Meyhoffer says: "Nit. ac., 3× and 6× in great irritation, redness and ulceration of the epiglottis and larynx, with difficult and painful deglutition, violent dry cough and nocturnal perspiration. The inhalation of 5 or 10 drops of the first dilution to an ounce of water, has mitigated rapidly the troublesome throat symptoms in tubercular laryngitis." In syphilitic laryngitis, with hoarseness, aphonia, ulceration of the buccal mucous membrane, complete obstruction of the nose, or fetid yellow discharge, with an inflamed and swollen nose; coryza; dry cough, etc., Nit. ac. is well nigh a specific." Dr. Holcomb says: "Nit. ac., 1st centesimal trituration, frequently succeeds with those obstinate, dry coughs, after Atropine has failed."

Dr. Bayes says: "Nit. ac. is indicated in specific ulcerations of mucous surfaces, using 3rd dilution, but changing to lower forms if a favorable change does not speedily supervene; also in a certain form of chronic laryngeal cough, dry, with a stinging or smarting sensation, as if from a small ulcer, generally felt on one side."

Aggravations, in the evening by deep breathing, reading aloud or talking, damp, cold air, or getting wet.

NUX VOMICA (DRY) — Very irritable and given to scolding; symptoms aggravated early in the morning, about 3 A.M.; suffers much from dyspepsia, especially those that live high, or take intoxicating liquors; greatly troubled with an acid stomach,

> constipation and frequently with hæmorrhoids; much flatulent colic, with ineffectual urging to stool; dry, racking cough, with great soreness of the stomach.

Cough that is curable with Nux vomica is of recent origin, of a dry scraping character, and not founded on an organic base, but of a simple catarrhal nature, or of a reflex character, from the digestive organs, or spinal. Dr. Hirschel says: "Nux vomica has only a limited application in cough, especially where the pharynx and fauces are affected. The cough is scraping, rough, with irritation in the throat or under the upper sternal parts, with difficult expectoration of tough mucus, on awakening from sleep in the morning, renewed or aggravated by vomiting and eating. Dry coryza, influenza, or general simple catarrhs."

Dr. Baehr has no faith in this remedy in acute bronchitis and pneumonia; but in chronic bronchitis he has some confidence in it, he says: "If the cough sets in with a particular violence between midnight and morning, is dry, spasmodic, very persistent and racking, so as to cause pain in the bowels, is easily excited by a change of temperature, and is associated with a continual titillation in the chest and trachea; only in the morning, mostly after, very seldom before rising, a loose cough sets in, with easy expectoration of a simple mucus. While coughing a sensation of soreness and roughness is sensibly felt down the middle of the chest. The condition of the digestive organs greatly facilitates the selection of the right remedy. In contradistinction to Sulphur, Nux vomica is much better adapted to comparatively recent cases without any serious complications, and otherwise more particularly suitable for patients with vigorous and otherwise sound constitutions."

Aggravations—After midnight and early in the morning; in the open air; by becoming cold; from motion and vexation.

COUGH

Relieved from warm air and warmth in general; in damp, wet weather and from lying down.

> **OPIUM (DRY)** — Dry, teasing, titillating cough, day and night, but especially at night; cough of a cerebral origin, especially fright; face swollen and purple with soporous sleep and stertorous breathing; constipation, stools composed of round, hard, black balls; much perspiration that is cold and clammy; bed feels so hard he cannot lie upon it; frequent hot flushes. No pains are found in the Opium cough.

For a dry, spasmodic, teasing, titillating cough aggravated at night, of a cerebro-spinal origin, Opium will be found of great value, but if deep organic changes have taken place another remedy will have to be selected.

Dr. Hirschel says: "Opium—Spasmodic cough with a continuous dry, titillation, allowing no rest either by day or night. In every other case, as in the cough of phthisical patients, where it keeps off nightly paroxysms, it acts only palliatively by it's *narcotic* quality; but for such a purpose strong allopathic doses are necessary."

Baehr says: "Never give Opium in cough with profuse expectoration of mucus, or it will tend to great dryness."

"The desire to cough is follwed immediately by an arrest of respiration and a blue face."—*Guernsey*.

In the treatment of chronic bronchitis Baehr says: "It is erroneous to suppose that the narcotic effect of Opium suspends the desire to cough only for a short time, for there are many forms of cough where Opium only aggravates, and does not afford any relief, or affords relief only when administered in very large doses, to be followed afterwards by an increase in the cough. In our opinion, Opium is admirably homœopathic to a spasmodic, dry, paroxysmal, titillating cough, which is especially tormenting at night and has but a scanty expectoration. The fact that we have often cured a cough of this kind permanently by means of a few doses of Opium, entitles us to the belief that Opium is something better than a mere palliative in this affection. In the later course of tuberculosis, after suppuration had really set in, we have obtained speedy and real relief by means of small doses of *Morphine*, one-twentieth, or one-fiftieth of a grain at a dose, nor have we ever hesitated to avail ourselves of the narcotic properties of this agent."

Where Opium is indicated there is no pain attending the disease.

Aggravations from brandy; anxiety; during sleep and especially at night.

PHOSPHORUS (DRY) — This is truly a lung remedy and affects more favorably slender people with fair skin, sanguine temperament and a very sensitive disposition; deep seated organic diseases, where death is inevitable; sensation of weakness and emptiness in the abdomen; this distresses and aggravates all the other symptoms, and is the ruling key for the use of Phosphorus. Stools, slim, hard and dry, evacuated with great difficulty, looking like a dog's; diarrhea, which pours out in great quantities like water from a hydrant, with a weak, all gone sensation in the whole abdominal cavity; hard, tight, rough, short, dry cough; heat or burning in the back between the shoulders; obstinate, profuse hæmorhages; cold feet and legs; cold, clammy sweats; emaciated people, who take cold very easily and are very sensitive to cool air.

For deep seated organic affections of the air passages, with a rough, short, tight, dry cough, Phosphorus is of an inestimable value. Dr. Hirschel says: "The indications for Phosphorus in nervous cough are similar to Opium, and may also be compared with Belladonna and Drosera. In Opium one might say the titillation is the chief indication; in Phos., the cough is more tormenting. The irritation from Phosphorus is not so continuous as that of Opium. In Belladonna, also, the cough is more mild—not so deeply seated. The similarity with Drosera consists in this,—that in both the cough comes in paroxysms with intervals. The cough in Phos. is cut off short; cough, short, dry; between every single coughing sound is a short interval, which is wanting in the Drosera cough, where they follow one another in quick succession; the cough does not begin with deep inspiration, but the expiration prevails; the patient keeps coughing when lying down, without any necessity to sit up for it, and the fit does not terminate with expectoration or vomiting of mucus, but ceases gradually. Neither does the Phosphorus cough come so apparently from the depth of the abdomen; the patients rather point to the upper or lower respiratory organs (larynx, bronchi, lungs). It is quite certain that in such nervous coughs Phosphorus is a grand remedy, hence it's splendid effects in stenosis of the glottis, in coughs from bronchial asthma, in angina pectoris (carbiac cough). Phosphorus is of an equally great value in catarrhal, inflammatory, or organic diseases of the respiratory organs. We find it everywhere in laryngeal, tracheal, bronchial, pulmonary catarrh up to inflammation, even in the most croupous form, or terminating in pseudo-plasmata and disorganization of the tissue. The painfulness of the larynx to touch; the different pains, soreness, stitches, burning; the expectoration of foamy, sticky, purulent, salty, sweetish, brown, rust coloured, bloody mucus; the cough is aggravated by speaking, laughing, eating, motion; hoarseness and aphonia; shortness of breath and orthopnea; great debility and prostration, the fever—all of them prove the deeply penetrating action of this remedy, still showing it's power in emphysema and tuberculosis. In a fit of coughing during measles, where the child for twelve hours steadily felt an irritation to cough, and expectorated a little foam and blood, after all other remedies failed; a single dose of Phos. 2 stopped it permanently. In pneumonia it always remains our sheet-anchor, and it prevents in croup, paralysis and narcosis through the carbonized blood."

C.C. Smith says: "Phosphorus—Goneness in the region of the stomach; hoarseness and aphonia in the evening; tormenting cough, tight and worse before midnight; painless diarrhea; puffiness around the eyes; night sweat, especially during sleep; cough worse from eating and drinking; cough, with a bursting sensation in the head; aphthous patches at the roof of mouth and tongue."

"Especially when there is sensitiveness and dryness of the larynx, with a feeling as if it was lined with fur and an inability to utter a word, every effort to do so being painful; nervous exhaustion; suspected atrophy of nerve tissues."—*W. H. Holcomb, M.D.*

Baehr says: "Phosphorus, according to our own experience is less adapted to phthisis as a whole than to single symptoms. It has to be used with caution, for no other medicine causes hæmoptysis as easily as Phosphorus. No other medicine disagrees so completely in the long run. The chief indications for Phosphorus are : continued hoarseness, with a distressing, dry cough, sore feeling in the larynx and trachea; pain in the stomach after every meal; also retching and vomiting of mucus; continuous diarrhea, which is excited by eating, and after every meal; excessive excitement of sexual passion."

Meyhoffer says: "Phosphorus will rarely benefit the chronic catarrh of persons otherwise healthy; but it is admirably suited to the intercurrent acute or subacute attacks of bronchitis in emaciated, cachectic or young, overgrown invalids. The tendency to pulmonary congestion and catarrhal pneumonia, so often, under such circumstances, either the proximate cause or complication of bronchial irritation, are additional and important indications for Phosphorus. It is also one of our chief remedies in broncho-pulmonary catarrh resulting from dilatation or fatty degeneration of the heart. I am as yet unable to give an opinion as to the dose, the 3rd and 30th having served me equally well."

Dr. T. Nichol says: "Phosphorus is the principal remedy in bronchitis of any kind, when the inflammatory irritation threatens to attack the parenchyma of the lungs, and it is customary to administer it after the more acute symptoms have been subdued by Aconite. The cough is dry and hacking, with burning and tickling in the air passages, and stitches in the chest. It is aggravated by speaking, laughing or drinking, and is followed by expectoration of a bloody and frothy mucus. There is also painful sensitiveness of the larynx, with hoarseness or complete aphonia. The respiration is loud and panting, indicative of great oppression, and the pulse is hard and hurried, or rapid and feeble. Phosphorus seems useful in almost any dilution, but the 6th to the 12th seem to be the most successful."

"In incipient as well as confirmed phthisis, in persons of meagre, slender form, fair complexion, and strong sexual feelings; when in the lower lobes and of an asthenic type, in children and young people (girls) of delicate constitutions, with dry, short cough, shortness of breath, great emaciation, tendency to diarrhea, or perspiration, it is useful. It is not specific for phthisis, but acts usefully on certain states of lowered nervous energy."

"Violent pneumonia with sticking pains in the chest, excited or aggravated by coughing or breathing, also in pleuro-pneumonia, when they are violent and extend over a large surface; when a large portion of the lung is inflamed, with dyspnea, the cough is dry, and the sputa *rust coloured.* Phosphorus is in many cases the only remedy, and it affords relief in four or eight hours. Give three drops of the third dilution every two or three hours."

"Where the cough is not so loose and rattling as in Lycopodium, or so close and tight as in Bryonia, the secretion also being of a more *dirty appearnce resembling pus but thinner, and when falling on any hard, smooth surface will break and fly like thin batter,* Phosphorus 30th or 200th will remove the whole trouble with remarkable promptness." —*C.Pearson, M.D.*

Aggravations, cough day and night, but especially at night; from cold air, or from change of weather; and from motion or laughing.

Relieved by warm air; in the dark and after sleeping.

> **PULSATILLA PRATENSIS (MOIST)** — Very affectionate females with blue eyes, yielding disposition and easily excited to tears; symptoms aggravate in a close, warm room; craves fresh, cool air; symptoms very changeable, well one hour and sick the next; especially affects the posterior spinal nerves; has constant chillness, coldness and paleness of the skin; weeps very easily, can hardly give her symptoms without weeping; always has a very bad taste in the morning with thickly coated, white or yellow tongue; sour stomach, from the least digression in diet, especially bad effects from rich, fat food; inclined to mucous diarrhea, worse at night; women that are inclined to be fleshy, with delayed and scanty menstruation; loose, rattling, hard, racking cough, that makes the stomach sore, and emissions of urine at every paroxysm of coughing.

This is a grand remedy for the second stage of catarrhal coughs, not depending on an organic base, the cough is loose, with copious mucous expectoration, accompanied with great soreness of the epigastric region, and if in a female, urine is emitted at each cough. It is apt to be very loose through the day and tight at night.

Dr. Hirschel says: "Pulsatilla is similar to Hepar; when given too early, even in the third dilution, it will produce aggravation and render the cough dry after resolution sets in. Pulsatilla, like Hepar, suits only moist cough with copious mucous expectoration especially when yellow, whitish, salty, towards the end of catarrhs, or in chronic catarrhs. Pulsatilla encroaches not so deeply upon the metamorphosis as Hepar, and is, therefore, only a palliative in chronic organic cases. It is especially indicated for mucous rales, where asthmatic disturbances arise from the accumulation of phlegm (emphysema), with catarrhal irritation in the throat; amelioration in fresh air; aggravation in the evening and at night. It is a specific in those cases where the cough is moist during the day, with a dry, titillating cough at night in a recumbent position."

"What could we do without *Pulsatilla* in presence of copious muco-purulent expectoration in lymphatic and anæmic females? There is no remedy which corresponds so well with the irregularities of function in the reproductive organs, as well as with the symptomatology of the bronchial affection, so common to this class of women, as the *meadow anemone*. Nocturnal paroxysms of dyspnea, gouty or rheumatic pains, flying about from one part of the body to another, worse at night, fix as characteristic symptoms to the selection of this remedy. I never used a higher dilution than the 3d."—*Mayhoffer*.

Dr. T. Nichol says: "Pulsatilla is the leading remedy when an attack of acute bronchitis threatens to assume a chronic form."

"Pulsatilla is much more useful in chronic than in acute bronchitis, if the following symptoms prevail: cough, principally at night, excited by itching in the trachea, with copious expectoration of mucus; the mucus is mostly white, but frequently mingled with yellowish or greenish lumps that impart to it an oily, offensive taste. There must not be any emphysema, whereas the presence of tubercles as the cause of the disease points to Pulsatilla. Pulsatilla is next to indispensable in bronchial catarrh of chlorotic patients which almost always, although not in every case, depends upon tubercles. If in the case of children, an acute catarrh gradually changes to the chronic form, Pulsatilla is a remedy of the first importance." *Baehr.*

The cough of Pulsatilla is at first dry, but it subsequently becomes moist, with considerable expectoration of a saltish or bitterish phlegm, or of phlegm tinged with blood, or of a yellowish or whitish appearance. The cough is attended with stitches and pain in the chest, with soreness of the throat and palate, and it proceeds from a tickling or an itching in the larynx; or by a scraping dryness in the trachea, accompanied with fatiguing pains in the abdomen and stitches in the back, shoulders, side or chest. It is relieved by rising up in bed. The racking cough exacerbates at night and in a recumbent position. It is accompanied by rattling of phlegm, nausea, or even vomiting, and sensation of being stifled, with a feeling of soreness or contusion about the belly, in the act of coughing. Hoarseness or even complete aphonia may be present and coryza with a yellowish, greenish and fetid discharge is not rare.

Marcy advises the 1st to the 6th potency, but I have seen the best results from dilutions ranging from the 12th to the 30th.

Aggravations, evening till midnight; from warmth, especially in a warm, close room; from lying down; from fatty rich food and from tobacco smoke.

Relieved, in the open air; by cold air and in a cool place; by cold drinks; with head high and by walking.

RHUS TOXICODENDRON (DRY) — Coughs brought on by cold damp weather; patient cannot lie long in one position, has to shift about constantly to obtain relief, which lasts but a short time, when he has to move again; patient always gets worse after midnight; great stiffness of the limbs before a storm; great lameness and stiffness, pain on first moving after rest; relieved by continued motion; fiery red tongue; putrid taste, after the first mouthful; has no appetite; looseness of the bowels, worse at night, with great exhaustion; involuntary stools; cough brought on by repeated drenchings in the rain; terrible cough, which seems as if it would tear something out of the chest; brick dust expectoration, raised with great difficulty; vesicular eruptions on the skin, with erysipelas.

For acute cases of cough, with much prostration of the whole system and for dry, racking, hard, rheumatic coughs, greatly aggravated at night, Rhus t. will be found of great value. The case is apt to take on a low typhoid form, where Rhus t. is indicated.

"Rhus is in it's place if the local affection is so disguised by the constitutional disease that we seem to be dealing with typhus complicated with bronchial catarrh. The use of the remedy is suggested by great debility, a prostrated condition of the whole organism, symptoms of violent reaction, such as a rapid pulse, burning heat, dry skin and tongue, delirium, mostly at night, excited by motion and by every little cold current of air; tickling and a feeling of dryness in the throat, down the trachea; the symptoms abate for awhile after a swallow of warm water or tea, but soon reappears in the same degree, accompanied by tearing pains in the extremities, especially if they set in at the same time as the cough, in consequence of the patient being exposed to the influence of a damp and cold air, or getting soaking wet; the paroxysms occur at night, attended with complete sleeplessness; the cough is complicated with coryza and frequent spasmodic sneezing, or in a case of influenza, with typhoid symptoms."—*Baehr.*

"Rhus t.—Worse in the evening, at night and with perfect rest. Symptoms lessened by rising from the bed and walking about. On the other hand they are aggravated by external cold, while frictions and warm application relieve them. Though gentle exercise relieves them, they are aggravated by all rough movements or severe exertions."—*Marcy and Hunt.*

"Acute catarrh; the nasal, laryngeal, tracheal and bronchial passages seem stuffed up; commencing at about sunset with sneezing and a dry, hard, tickling cough; very severe, continuing until midnight, when all the sufferings are relieved; renewed next morning."—*Dr. Boyce.*

In pneumonia, expectoration of brick dust or bloody sputa, raised with great difficulty; accompanied with low typhoid symptoms.

Aggravations, by cold bathings or getting drenched with rain; in cold, damp weather; from taking cold after being heated. In the evening, until midnight, the cough is quickly aggravated by cold air, or uncovering a single part of the body, a hand or foot, and by drinking cold water or beer.

Relieved, by warm air and after having moved awhile.

RUMEX CRISPUS (DRY) — Especially acts upon the mucous membrane of the larynx and trachea. Violent and incessant, dry, fatiguing cough, with little expectoration, aggravated by pressure, talking, especially inspiring cool air and at night; cannot bear the cold air, covers up the head to exclude it; sense of excoriation behind the sternum; complete aphonia.

COUGH

This remedy has a powerful and specific action upon the larynx and trachea, and for dry, hard, teasing, nocturnal cough, that is greatly excited and aggravated by cool air, Rumex will give the most complete satisfaction. I cannot refrain from giving the precise and practical remarks of Dr. C. Dunham in this remedy. He says: "I have used Rumex chiefly in acute catarrhal affections of the larynx, trachea and bronchi. In these cases it seems to present a close analogy in it's action to Belladonna, Lachesis, Phosphorus and Causticum. Rumex diminishes the secretions and at the same time exalts in a very marked manner the sensibility of the mucous membrane of the larynx and trachea, exceeding in the extent of this exaltation any remedy known to us. The cough, therefore, is frequent and continuous, to an extent quite out of proportion to the degree of organic affection of the mucous membrane. It is dry, occurs in long paroxysms, or, under certain circumstances, is almost uninterrupted. It is induced, or greatly aggravated, by any irregularity of respiration, such as an inspiration of air a little colder than that previously inhaled; by irregularity of respiration and motion of the larynx and trachea, such as are involved in the act of speech, and by external pressure upon the trachea in the region of the supra-sternal fossa. The subjective symptoms are : rawness and soreness in the trachea, extending a short distance below the supra-sternal fossa and laterally into the bronchi, chiefly the left; and tickling in the supra-sternal fossa and behind the sternum, provoking the cough; this tickling is very annoying and very persistent, is often but momentarily, and sometimes only partially relieved by coughing. The cough occurs chiefly, or is much worse in the evening after retiring, and at the time the membrane of the trachea is particularly sensitive to cool air and to any irregularity in the flow of air over it's surface, so that the patient often covers the head with bed clothes to avoid the cold air of the apartment, and refuses to speak, or even to listen to conversation, for fear his attention should be withdrawn from the supervision of his respiratory acts, which he performs with the most careful uniformity and deliberation, and all in the hope of preventing the distressing tickling and the harassing cough which would ensue from a neglect of these precautions. I have frequently witnessed this state of things during the last three years, and have invariably given prompt relief with Rumex. In the group of remedies in which I have placed Rumex (along with Bell., Lach., Phos. and Caust.), it stands pre-eminent in respect to the extreme sensibility of the tracheal mucous membrane. All of these remedies produce symptoms identical in kind; the characteristic of each is to be found in the relative degree in which each symptom is pronounced in the different remedies, quite as much as in the possession by any one of them of symptoms not produced by others. Thus Bell., Lach. and Rumex, each produce a dry cough, induced by tickling in the larynx or trachea, and provoked by deep inspiration, speaking and by external pressure on the larynx or trachea. The cough of each is spasmodic and long continued, and is worse at night after retiring; but apart from the fact that Bell. and Lach. act more upon the lower part of the trachea, we observe that in the case of Lach. the slightest external pressure on the larynx or trachea produces violent and long continued spasmodic cough; the patient cannot endure the least constriction in that region, not even the ordinary contact of his clothing. There is, moreover a sense of fullness in the trachea and a long painful aching in the whole extent of the os hyoides. In the case of Bell., not only is cough produced to a moderate extent by pressing upon the larynx, but soreness and pain are experienced, with a sense of internal fullness and soreness, which at once suggests the presence of acute laryngitis sub-mucosa. In Rumex on the other hand, there is no sensibility, strictly speaking, of the trachea, but simply such an instability of the mucous membrane that cough is produced by the change of position induced in that membrane by external pressure on the trachea. As regards the extent and intensity of this symptom, Rumex holds a lower rank than the other remedies named. But the irritability of the mucous membrane, by virtue of which cough is induced by hurried or deep inspiration, or by speaking, while it is common to Bell., Lach., Rumex and Phosphorus, is produced in the most exalted degree, as we have already seen, by Rumex, which, as regards this symptom, takes the first rank. A sensation of rawness or roughness in the larynx, trachea and bronchi is produced by each of the four remedies, but the *locality* and the *degree* in which it is produced, vary in such a manner as to serve in some measure as a characteristic of each. It is most marked in Phos. and Bell., less prominent in Rumex, and least of all in Lach. In Bell. and Lach. it is most marked in the larynx; indeed, it is almost confined to that region. Rumex produces it in the trachea and upper part of the bronchi, while Phos. induces it in the whole mucous tract, from the larynx to the small bronchioles, and in the Phosphorus proving this rawness of the air passages is accompanied by a no less characteristic sense of weight and constriction across the upper part of the thorax, which indicates an affection of the finer air tubes, and of the air vesicles, of such a character as seriously to impede the function of respiration. In considering this last symptom we must mention Causticum also, which produces rawness, extending along the whole length of the sternum. All five remedies produce hoarseness; Phosphorus causing, Causticum and Bell., most eminently, Rumex less decidedly and Lachesis in a still lesser degree."

Aggravations in the evening after lying down; by pressure upon the larynx and trachea and especially by the inhalation of cool air; patient often covers up the head with the bed clothes to avoid inhaling the cool air of the bed room.

Relieved by warm air.

> **SANGUINARIA CANADENSIS (MOIST)** — Cough that has passed into the second stage and the lungs are filled with mucus, raised with difficulty; rusty coloured sputa in the second stage of pneumonia; excessive dyspnea; cough with coryza, then diarrhea; constitutional and severe cough, with or without expectoration, always attended with circumscribed redness of the cheeks; croup, membrane difficult to detach; constant and incessant dry cough on lying down at night, relieved by sitting up.

This is a precious remedy for cough, either in the subacute, or chronic form, where the larger bronchial tubes are involved, and the stage of mucous secretion has been reached. The cough sounds very loose, but the mucus is expectorated with difficulty.

Dr. Holcomb says : "I prescribe it in a certain troublesome, harassing cough without a marked inflamatory action, when you are uncertain about whether you are dealing with a chronic bronchitis or an incipient tuberculosis, I use the 1st centesimal trituration of the resenoid. I have been astonished at the power of this remedy in such cases. It has done me more good in pulmonary diseases than any other single remedy. Calcarea 200, one powder before breakfast and one powder of Sanguinaria 1st an hour or two after each meal, for chronic bronchial diseases, has procured me more reputation and business, than any other one prescription I have ever made." In moist cough he says: "Sanguinaria, 3d centesimal trituration steadily persisted for several days, will arrest this catarrhal disease in almost any of it's forms, although when there is headache, sore throat, red cheeks, pains in the breast, offensive breath and expectoration; or symptoms threatening, it proves of very great efficacy."

Dr. C.C. Smith says: "Sanguinaria—Emptiness of stomach, worse after eating, a flushed face, followed by hectic spots upon cheeks; constant tickling at the entrance of larynx, causing a constant cough, with a crawling sensation down behind the sternum; chest sore and painful to touch; hot streamings from chest to abdomen; cold hands and blue nails; breath and sputa offensive even to the patient; extreme dyspnea; desire to take a deep breath, which is followed by intense pain on the right side of chest, lassitude in the mornings, aversion to motion; stools predominantly loose; cough relieved by passage of flatus upward or downward; syphilitic patients."

In pseudo-membranous bronchitis, Dr. T. Nichol places this remedy next to Kalium bichromicum, and finds it difficult to give the differential diagnosis between the two remedies. "When the sibilant rale predominates and the faint and almost absent mucous rale shows that the pseudo-membrane is closely adherent to the wall of the bronchial tubes, Sanguinaria should be given; should the sibilant rale be less violent and the mucous rale indicates a less tenacious membrane, Kali bi. is in place. Both remedies should be given in material doses, for the high dilutions are veritably *hgh delusions* here."

Marcy and Hunt say: "This is one of the best agents we have for the prevention, if not the cure of consumption. We have used it with success in patients who were subject to distressing affections of the chest, repeated attacks of pneumonia, hæmoptysis and spasmodic attacks resembling pertussis. Also in protracted catarrhal fever, which leaves obstinate cough and threatening consumption. The cough has generally been mitigated, the pulse diminished in frequency and the powers of the whole digestive system increased; the appetite is always improved, or regulated in cases where it has been morbidly great. Chronic dryness in the throat; continuous, severe dry cough, with pain in the chest and circumscribed redness of the cheeks; tormenting cough with expectoration. The peculiar cough, emaciation and hectic fever of pulmonary consumption; hydrothorax, asthma, pneumonia and pneumonia typhoides, pain in the chest, with cough and expectoration; burning and pressing in the breast and back; palpitations of the heart; burning of the palms of the hands and soles of the feet at night."

"Sanguinaria, has also like *Phos.* a feeling of emptiness or *goneness* in the region of the stomach, but it occurs particularly *after eating*. Flashes of heat on the face similar to *Sulphur,* but leaving behind them circumscribed red spots on the cheeks similar to hectic. Constant *tickling* at the *entrance* of the *larynx* causing a *continuous* cough, which is worse in the *evening,* on *lying down,* with a crawling sensation extending down beneath the *sternum;* chest sore and *painful* to the touch (Calc.); sensation of *hot steam* passing from the *chest* to the *abdomen, cold hands* and *blue nails.* The *breath* and *sputa* smell *badly* even to the patient; *dyspnea extreme;* disposition to take a *long breath,* which is followed by intense pain in the *right side* of chest. *Great lassitude,* especially in the *evening;* does not want to move or make any mental exertion; stools *predominantly loose.* The cough is relieved by passing flatus *upwards* and *downwards.* Sanguinaria should be thought of *first,* perhaps, in phthisis occurring in syphilitic patient."—*C. C. Smith, M. D.*

SENEGA (MOIST) — Profuse secretion of mucus in the lungs with loose, rattling cough; hydrothorax, ascites and anasarca; sensation of trembling, with no visible trembling; great burning in the chest, either before or after coughing; much pain and soreness in the chest, worse during rest.

"Senega has great power of aiding the expectoration of tough phlegm in torpid states of the laryngeal and bronchial mucous membrane, as we find in old persons; in lax phlegmatic constitutions and in chronic catarrhal difficulties, in emphysema, in senile asthma, in bronchiectasis and in tuberculosis. It aids in removing the catarrh with long continued coughing spells, or where the hepatization of acute pneumonia, resolution is tardy, on in chronic cases with cheesy infiltration."—*Dr. Hirschel.*

"Constant accumulation of phlegm in the bronchial tubes with irritation in the bowels, tending to diarrhea; the irritation may alternate from the chest to the bowels and *vice versa.*"—*F. W. Ingles, M. D.*

"Twentieth day of pneumonia in a woman at fifty six, right side, violent stiches, sinking of strength, small, scarcely perceptible pulse, short, rare cough, without expectoration, great rattling of mucus in the chest, somnolence, dejected features. After the second dose of *Senega*, expectoration began and recovery took place. In the same place it was also recorded that a parish doctor had saved the lives of about one hundred patients affected with adynamic pneumonia, with *Senega*. It is also said to be an excellent remedy in the mucoid cough of old people who bring up a great quantity of watery mucus."—*Dr. Hallenbach.*

"Senega has no small merit when, in copious accumulation of mucus in the air tube, the latter causes by it's adhesiveness to all the organs through which it's passage lies the greatest, often the most ineffectual, efforts of coughing and hawking for it's expulsion."—*Dr. Meyhoffer.*

Aggravated, in the evening and at night, during rest, in a warm room.

Relieved in cool air.

SEPIA OFFICINALIS (DRY) — Putrid urine, it cannot be suffered to remain in the room; the urine deposits a reddish, clay coloured sediment, which adheres to the bottom and sides of the vessel as if it was burned on. In women, sensation as if everything would come out of the vagina; she has to cross her limbs to prevent it; constipation, stools hard, difficult and knotty, with a sense of weight in the anus, not relieved at stool; yellow saddle across the nose; acts more favorably upon the female sex, especially if complicated with ovario-uterine disease.

To me this is a difficult remedy to select in cough, it being useful in either dry or loose cough. In my opinion the dry cough predominates, and it acts much better in females than it does in males. Dr. Hirschel says: "The provings of Sepia show dry and moist cough, even copious expectoration of white, salted mucus or pus. I find it effectual in that dry cough which is so characteristic of tuberculosis. We find titillation in the trachea, sometimes a covered, deep voice without timbre, sensation of dryness in the chest or throat, dry, croaking, deep cough, somewhat ameliorated when lying down. After great labor some mucus may be expectorated, which is tough, slimy or albuminous. Next to Calcarea, Sepia is for me a chief remedy in tuberculosis. I also use it successfully in chronic catarrhs, especially when they are complicated with chronic gastric catarrh, or when venous stasis is present. Taking all in all the action of Sepia is less extensive, and its selection must be well studied."

Kreusler says that "Sepia will be found applicable to chronic inflammation of the air passages, if psora be a complicating element", and Meyhoffer thinks that its indication will be apparent when the totality of symptoms forbids the exhibition of Pulsatilla, and herpetic manifestations on the skin decidedly point towards the use of Sepia. "Sepia may claim our attention in a cough similar to Spongia, but we must confess that we have never derived very striking results from its use. The numerous symptoms in the pathogenesis of Sepia, which point to bronchial catarrh, give evidence that Sepia must be a remedy for this disease. Only it is dificult, owing to the multitude of symptoms, to present a characteristic group."—*Baehr.*

"The cough of Sepia is sometimes dry and spasmodic, attended with nausea and resulting in bilious vomiting, but is generally accompanied with abundant expectoration of greenish or yellowish matter, purulent or even bloody, and of a putrid or saltish taste. The cough exacerbates in the evening, also in the late evening hours, accompanied by soreness and weakness of the chest. A marked degree of dyspnea is present. Baehr points out that Sepia is not adapted to bronchial catarrhs, accompanied with bronchiectasis, emphysema, etc. Sepia acts best in the 30th dilution, and I have had fine results from the 12th trituration."—*Dr. T. Nichol.*

Aggravations, forenoon and evening until midnight, from cold damp north-east winds, and from repose.

Relieved in warm, dry air.

In chronic cough, Sepia follows well after Pulsatilla.

SILICEA TERRA (MOIST) — Deep seated organic coughs; where the nutrition of the tissue is assailed; great lack of vitality, cannot keep warm even when walking; great disposition to take cold, even from the slightest draft of air; tendency to suppuration, has wonderful power over suppuration, much perspiration upon the head and chest; children with large open fontanelles and who wish the head covered up; rachitis, with slow dentition. In women, great coldness during menstruation; constipation; stools difficult, as if the rectum did not have the power to expel them; the stool recedes after having been partially expelled; profuse, very fetid foot sweat; debilitating night sweats, etc.; caries of bones; fistulous ulcerations; excessive debility.

No remedy in the *materia medica* controls the suppurative process equal to Silicea. In organic diseases of the air passages, where suppuration has taken place, with a suffocative, racking, loose cough, copious expectoration of thick, yellow, greenish pus, hectic fever, great debility and profuse night sweats, this remedy will be our sheet anchor.

Dr. T. Nichol says : "Silicea is particularly suitable for lymphatic or sanguine individuals, and as a remedy for chronic bronchitis, it is only second to Sulphur."

Meyhoffer says: "I think it hardly possible to overcome radically the catarrh pituiteux of Laennec without the intervention of Silicea. In this form of bronchial disease no other agent contributes so largely towards recovery. Not less beneficial are the effects of Silicea in bronchial affections of rachitic children." Hughes thinks that Silicea may find its place in chronic bronchitis with puriform expectoration, while Teste coldly says: "Silicea is recommended in chronic bronchitis." Silicea is one of the principal remedies in obstinate or severe cases, characterized by a racking cough, with copious expectoration of a transparent purulent matter. The cough is suffocative with oppression of the chest, is aggravted at night, and is sometimes accompanied by a sore throat, with loss of breath when lying on the back and when stooping. All unite in prescribing the higher dilutions. Baehr says that "we have never derived any advantage from alcoholic attenuations, but always from the higher triturations."

Marcy and Hunt say : "This remedy embraces most of the symptoms that belong to the phthisical dyscrasia, consequently it is a remedy of value for the constitutional condition in congenital or hereditary cases. The dyspeptic symptoms peculiar to consumption are also nearly the same as under Hepar. The symptoms that show themselves in the larynx, with dry hacking cough, causing soreness in the chest; hoarseness with cough, suffocative night cough; excessive, continuous cough, with discharge of a translucent or bloody mucus; vomiting of purulent matter when coughing, ulceration of the lungs, discharge of clear, pure blood, with a deep, hollow cough; the chest is painful as if bruised; shortness of breath felt on walking or exercising; weakness and oppression of the chest, with chilliness of the surface; oppressive heaviness in the region of the heart and palpitations when sitting still."

Aggravations, in the evening and at night; from cold air, from any single part of the body becoming cold; getting cold after sweating; change of temperature before a thunder storm.

Relieved in warm air or a warm room.

SPONGIA TOSTA (DRY) — Especially affects the larynx and trachea; dry, hard, tight, hollow, croupy cough; great hoarseness; loss of voice; great dryness of the larynx; with hoarse, hollow wheezing cough; symptoms aggravated by lying down with the head low; goitre.

Spongia corresponds to affections of the upper part of the respiratory organs, especially the larynx and trachea. The cough is croupy, dry, sibilant, sounding like a saw driven though a pine board, each cough corresponding to a thrust of the saw.

Beahr says: "Spongia is characterized by a hollow, barking, dry, seldom moist cough, continuing all day, and likewise all night, in long lasting distressing paroxysms; at the same time labored, crowing, wheezing inspirations, sometimes accompanied by rales. The remedy is most appropriate for children, more particularly if the disease sets in as laryngitis and gradually extended to the lungs. It is an excellent remedy in croupous bronchitis."

"Often the patient is quite convalescent, when on very slight exposure the cough returns with redoubled violence—the most pressing dyspnea, sibilant ronchi and violent convulsive cough. When this relapse occurs, Spongia is pre-eminently the remedy, even though it had not been previously indicated." *Dr. Nichol.*

The first inflammatory symptoms should be subdued by Aconite.

This remedy is not used as much as it ought to be in those hard, tough cases of what might be called *dry bronchitis*. There is an absence of inflammatory symptoms, but the patient has a terrible hard, dry, racking cough, slight expectoration and much dyspnea. The triturations will give the best satisfaction.

Aggravations at night from cold air, especially northeast wind; and lying with the head low.

Relieved by warm air.

STANNUM METALLICUM (MOIST) — Profound prostration of the cerebro-spinal nervous system; patient must drop down, but can get up very well; can go up stairs nicely, but coming down stairs produces great faintness; reading aloud or talking produces great exhaustion; great weakness of the legs, they are not able to support the body; pains commence lightly, increase gradually to a very high degree, and then decrease again as slowly; profuse greenish expectoration; bronchial dilatation, with profuse purulent expectoration. Exhausting night sweats.

In chronic bronchitis, where the mucous secretion is very copious, of greenish, yellow or purulent matter, with a loose, rattling cough, accompanied with excessive prostration, especially centering in the chest, Stannum will be found of great utility. "Rough throat, hoarseness, weakness and emptiness in the chest; the hoarseness was sometimes momentarily relieved by a fit of cough; mucus in the trachea, in the forenoon, easily thrown off by a slight cough, the chest feels very weak as if deadened all over, with faintness of the whole body and limbs, in which a weak feeling is moving up and down, many mornings in succession. Accumulation of mucus in the chest, with rattling breathing which can be felt internally and heard by others; titillating creeping in the throat (larynx), with a feeling of dryness, obliging one to cough; irritation in the trachea during an inspiration, as if from mucus, there being neither mucous nor dry cough; it is more violently felt when sitting crooked than when walking; short cough from time to time, as if from weakness of the chest, with hoarse, weak sound; short and hacking cough; constant desire to cough, as if owing to too much mucus in the chest, with an internal feeling of panting and slight rattling; constant desire to cough, from a continual constriction of the trachea; titillating cough, as if from soreness deep in the trachea, with scratching rising up into the throat; exhausting fits of cough, which produce a bruised sort of pain in the pit of the stomach; oppression of the chest when coughing; scraping in the throat, with greenish expectoration of a disagreeably sweetish taste, more violent in the evening before going to bed; hoarse speech; after every cough (with irritation in the lower part of the trachea) sore feeling in the chest and trachea; horrid cough, with expectoration and spitting of blood; yellow discharge from the trachea, having a putrid taste; salty expectoration; fit of asthma, short breathing and anguish in the evening, obliged to breathe hurriedly for a long time, until he succeeds in drawing a deep breath, when the shortness disappears."— *Hahnemann.*

Aggravations by rapid motion, reading aloud and at night.

SULPHUR (MOIST) — Constant heat on the top of the head; has happy dreams; everything looks pretty which the patient takes a fancy to; excoriation about the anus and vagina; morning diarrhea that drives the patient out of bed in great haste, can't wait, must go to stool as soon as the desire is felt; obstinate, chronic constipation, stools dark, hard and dry, expelled with great straining, accompanied with piles that bleed much; all the secretions are exceedingly acrid, and excoriating; very faint and weak at 11 A.M., cannot wait for dinner; chronic hæmorrhages; patient gets almost well when it returns again and again; great deal of burning in the palms of the hands and soles of the feet; hot flushes with faintness; patient feels suffocated, wants the doors and windows open; much rattling of mucus in the lungs; excessive sensitiveness of the skin, every trifling change in the temperature causes change in the temperature causes an exacerbation, even if the patient remains in his room; he is powerfully affected by changes in the weather.

This remedy is the back bone of our school, only a few diseases can be treated without its aid, and about all kinds of cough yield to its power, but particularly chronic bronchial catarrh, with excessive collection of mucus or muco-purulent matter, with loose, rattling cough and easy expectoration, especially during the day time. At night the mucus is more tenacious and raised with difficulty, but becomes easy in the morning. Baehr says: "Sulphur is utterly useless in phthisis, and cases where it has done good have been cases of chronic pneumonia."

In chronic bronchitis, he says: "Sulphur is undoubtedly the most important remedy we have in this disease, because it corresponds to the worst and most inveterate cases. If emphysema is present, this remedy may never yield any marked results; even its palliative effect is questionable. Brilliant results may, however, be obtained in cases of chronic catarrh of long standing, if the mucus is secreted in large quantities, or is very tenacious, and the symptoms point to a decided thickening of the mucous membrane. An eminent indication for Sulphur is the excessive sensitiveness of the skin, so that every trifling change of temperature causes an exacerbation, and that even if the patient remains in his room he is still powerfully affected by the changes in the weather. Only this hyperesthesia must not be caused by pulmonary tuberculosis; the tubercles atleast must not be in a state of suppuration. What we have said shows that the symptoms may be distinguished in two series. The cough is either loose, the mucus easily detached, but only at times, so that at night, for instance, there is a good deal of dry cough, whereas in the morning and during the day the cough is moist. The expectoration is mostly white, compact, but mixed with a number of yellowish or green lumps, showing that the mucus had been secreted in the bronchi for some time before being coughed up; it has a foul taste and even a bad odor, the accompanying hoarseness and sensation of rawness show that the larynx and trachea have become involved in the pathological process. Or else the cough sets in more violent paroxysms with considerable dyspnea, is dry and spasmodic, with wheezing in the chest; it occurs most generally late in the evening and at night, and it is only towards morning or after rising that tenacious glassy mucus is brought up after a slight coughing spell. The digestive symptoms and the condition of the liver, which generally appears very much enlarged in chronic catarrh, confirm the selection of Sulphur. It has always seemed to us that the triturations of Sulphur did not act as well in this disease as the attenuations prepared from the alcoholic tincture, and that, as a rule, higher potencies act better than the lower. Finally, we have to observe that in the case of decrepit, and more especially old individuals, Sulphur seldom does any good."

Dr. Hirschel says : "Sulphur allows a far more extensive application in chronic forms; less, perhaps, by its specific relations to cough than by its vasomotory effect, and by its power of causing a reaction in the metamorphosis. It acts favorably where the course of the disease is slow, without coming to any decision in acute cases, as in catarrh or inflammation (Sulphur effectually developes hepatizations), as well as in chronic diseases of the respiratory organs and of the heart. Sulphur shows in the proving all sorts of coughs and different expectorations, but the constitution of the patient and the adjective of the disease give us hints for its selection. Wherever a dyscrasia in on hand, the physician remembers Sulphur."

"Burning of feet at night, with a desire to uncover them; flushes of heat to the face; early morning diarrhea; cramps in claves of legs at night, or in feet while walking; sudden arrest of breathing while turning over in bed; better while sitting up; sensation as if the lungs touched the back while coughing; throat rough and dry, with burning; hoarseness in the morning."—*Dr. C.C. Smith.*

"Great desire to cough, but is partially suppressed; does not amount to a full, free cough; in whooping cough."—*Dr. W.H. Guernsey.*

"Complete aphonia, with hoarse, suffocating cough, and smarting in the chest. Sulphur 10 M cured in two days."—*Wm. H. Holcomb, M.D.*

"Sulphur—Dry cough with retching, vomiting and spasmodic constriction in the chest, chiefly in the evening, or at night when the patient is lying down; loose cough, with expectoration of profuse thick whitish or yellowish mucus, sometimes only during the day, with dry cough at night; obstinate dry cough, excited by tickling in the throat; lancinating pains in the chest and head; giddiness of sight when coughing; sensation of fullness in the chest, with oppression; rattling of mucus; palpitations of the heart."—*F.W. Ingalls, M.D.*

"Sulphur—This is perhaps the most perfect specific for phthisis in its unmixed psoric form, not only when it follows pneumonia, but also when the disease is hereditary, and in the period of purulent expectoration."

In cases of *incipient phthisis* it should only be given at long intervals, a single dose should be allowed to operate for several weeks undisturbed. Dr. Nuñes, of Madrid, says "he has cured some cases of confirmed phthisis by this remedy." Teste says, "if it has not cured phthisis, it has at least retarded it for several years."

Hahnemann regarded phthisis as a psoric disease and Sulphur as the first of *antipsoric* remedies. He refers to six cases in which consumption was caused by the repulsion of psora from the skin; later writers have admitted that Sulphur is a specific for itch, and also for the diseases caused by its recession.

Sulphur is specifically suited for phthisis in psoric constitutions, of a lymphatic temperament, subject to venous plethora and hæmorrhoids. There is a predisposition to take cold from the slight exposure, running into chronic catarrh; eruptions resembling those of scrofula appear on the skin; rheumatic pains without swelling; drawing pains in the limbs; unsteady gait and tremor of the hands; great general prostration; nervous exhaustion following debilitating losses; numbness of different parts, paralysis and emaciation; pains worse at night, relieved by external warmth; drowsiness and disturbed sleep; disturbing dreams; hallucinations and timidity.

The patient curable by Sulphur has generally some eruptive disease of the skin, or has had such affection (not necessarily the itch) repelled from the surface at some former time; he is subject to abscesses, boils, or swelling of the glands; hectic fever, followed by night sweats, or profuse sweat from slight heat or exercise. There is hypochondriacal sadness, disposition to weep; *irritated, taciturn* disposition; the head is dizzy;

intolerance of light. The face is pale, wan, blanched, sickly, bloated, with a wrinkled countenance; blue margins around the eyes; hepatic spots on the skin; swelling of gums; dryness of the tongue; favus on the skin. The throat is dry; mucoid expectoration; sore throat, vesicles on the surface; pressure in the throat as if from a lump; tonsils red, swollen; uvula enlarged; putrid taste in the morning, ravenous appetite or loss of appetite; acidity of stomach and sour eructations; heartburn, morning nausea, waterbrash and acid vomiting.

The stomach is painful on pressure; swelling, burning and cramp like contraction or spasm of the stomach; malaise before a meal, nausea after eating. Pain in the abdomen, with sensitiveness of the surface; spasmodic contractive colic, cutting pain and nausea, followed by diarrhea and tenesmus; hæmorrhoids, constipation with pain in the rectum as if it would protrude; mucous stools streaked with blood, passed with ascarides or lumbrici; strangury, fetid urine. The throat feels *rough*, the larynx dry, sore, it's sides swollen and feeling as if something lodged there. Hoarseness or loss of voice; catarrh, fluent coryza, rawness or spasmodic contraction of the chest; cough dry, short and hacking, and after a meal exciting retching or vomiting. At a later stage the cough is looser, raising thick mucous, then greenish masses; the cough excites violent headache, which in the occiput is pulsative; spitting of blood. The breathing is spasmodically arrested; asthma excited by a long or rapid walk, or ascending the stairs; suffocative paroxysms, especially coming on at night; talking causes a weak feeling in the chest; oppression, or contractive pain there; neuralgic stitches of the chest, extending to the sternum or back; palpitations of the heart, anxious throbbing with flushing of the face, or rush of blood to the head; leucorrhea. Irregular menstruation, cold hands and feet. It may not be proved that Sulphur has cured confirmed phthisis in advanced stages; but, says Teste: "There is no doubt, however, that serious affections of the air passages have frequently been arrested by it's use; affections which, without being tuberculous phthisis, would nevertheless have been equally fatal."—*Marcy and Hunt.*

"Cases that have been badly treated either with drugs, or which is very little better, by low attenuations, until hepatization or even abscess has followed, with pale, cold, damp skin, emaciation, hectic fever, swelling of the extremities, *purulent expectoration,* and a quick weak pulse."—*C. Pearson, M.D. U.S.M. Investigator, page 27, Vol. 1.*

The symptoms of Sulphur are so numerous and so contradictory that we will leave the physician to make out the balance by physiological induction and clinical experience.

Aggravation, afternoon to midnight; cold, damp weather; cold, or open cold air, and from getting warm in bed.

Relieved by heat; in dry weather and from drawing the limbs up.

> **TARTAR EMETIC (MOIST)** — Loose, rattling cough, which sounds as if there was a cupful of mucus in the lungs, and it was about to run over; large collection of mucus in the bronchial tubes, expectorated with great difficulty, from paralysis of the vagi; paralysis of the lungs with great dyspnea, and fits of suffocation: very great thirst day and night; cough and yawning consecutively.

This remedy is indicated when we have a very loose, rattling cough, the lungs seem loaded with mucus, but none is expectorated.

Dr. Hirschel says: "Tartar emetic—Cough *rattling;* it sounds loose without being loose; cough with vomiting of food after eating; stertorous tracheal and bronchial rattling. The rattling necessitates sitting up, with vomiting or dyspnea and fear of suffocation. In the teething cough of children, where we frequently hear the rattling from afar, which disappears after the paroxysms of cough. In pneumonia with high graded hepatization it aids expectoration when resolution begins to take place. In chronic bronchial catarrhs, emphysema, bronchiectasis, senile catarrhs. It gives great alleviation in tuberculosis pulmonum, but also more rapid dissolution of the tubercles, and hastens the downward course. In croup as an intermediate remedy for the solution, and to keep off paralysis. It acts well in those cases without producing emesis."

"Copious accumulation of mucus in the air passages, deficiency of aëration caused by it's presence, numerous moist rattles, severe spasmodic suffocative cough. *Tartar emetic* is *more adapted* to subacute than to chronic affections of the air tubes; hence it's frequent application in bronchial catarrh for children and aged persons. Infants especially, sometimes exhibit in the course of chronic bronchitis sudden and alarming symptoms of suffocation and mechanical irritation of the fauces is not always convenient or tolerated. In such cases a vomiting dose of this salt does much good and cannot do harm. A solution of one grain of the first decimal trituration to half an ounce of water, administered by teaspoonfuls every ten minutes, suffices to produce after the second or third dose, an ejection of the accumulated mucus. This proceeding is only to be adopted when a high degree of asphyxia demands immediate relief. Afterwards the 3d and 4th triturations act all the more favorably on the affected parts, as better oxidized blood contributes it's share to an improved nutrition of the bronchial lining."—*Meyhoffer.*

In capillary bronchitis, "*Tartar emetic* is unquestionably the great remedy for this dangerous form of bronchitis, and all who have used it can endorse the recommendation of Dr. Hughes: 'perfectly homœopathic to both the local and the general condition. I have almost invariably relied upon it single handed, and have seen desperate cases recover under it's use.' Kreussler says that he has 'found it very efficient in the last hours, when the patients struggled hard.' Baehr remarks that, 'it is really the second stage of the catarrhal process which is adapted to the curative action of this drug,' but my experience is that it should be given promptly and without delay, as soon as the disease is diagnosed. Aconite is the only remedy which can compare with it in value in this disease, and Aconite has almost always been given in the earlier stages of the malady. It is indicated by severe spasmodic suffocative cough, with wheezing respirations and marked dyspnea; also by a rattling cough which ends with vomiting of thick white mucus; also when the cough suddenly ceases, from weakness or from other causes. The actions of the patient seem to show that he is suffering from oppression at the chest, and the mucous ronchus, indicating a very copious accumulation of mucus in the bronchial tubes, is one of the leading features of the case. This accumulation forms a mechanical obstruction to respiration, and accordingly we have a group of symptoms of carbonic acid poisoning more or less pronounced, great anxiety and agitation, pale and bloated face, coma or delirium with coldness of the extremities. Profuse cool sweat not followed by relief, and a disposition to vomiting and diarrhea would be additional indications. The cough is aggravated by speaking, eating and the recumbent posture. Acts best in 3rd and 4th triturations."—*T. Nichol. M. D.*

Aggravations, in the evening; in damp, cold weather and from getting warm in bed.

Relieved, in the open, cold air.

> **VERATRUM ALBUM (DRY)** — The spasmodic element prevails in the cough. Cold sweat on the forehead; exhausting watery diarrhea, with cold sweat on the forehead; great desire for cold drings; great irritation of the cœliac plexus, with fainting, great prostration, nausea and vomiting and cold perspiration; asthma, with suffocation, blue face and anguish; second, or plastic stage of catarrh, with a loose rattling cough.

This is a special irritant to the vagus, and through it produces a hard, loose spasmodic cough, consequently is not called for until the second stage of catarrh has commenced.

Baehr says: "Veratrum album is not often enough made use of in bronchitis. It is not suitable in the first stage, but on the passage into the second stage, if mucus is secreted in copious quantities which cannot yet be coughed up. This causes a constant titillation deep in the chest, with a desire to cough; wheezing and coarse rales, but no expectoration; the depressing paroxysms of cough occurs principally at night, with violent determination of blood to the head. The general failing of strength, the increased frequency or even irregularity of the pulse constitute additional indications for Veratrum, which is evidently suitable to old people rather than children."

Hirschel says : "Just as Veratrum shows great similarity to Ipecac., in affections of the stomach and intestines, so also in cough. The titillation in Veratrum is only somewhat lower down, with a sensation of constriction in the throat; the oppression, the nausea, the vomiting of food and mucus is stronger after Veratrum, and the paroxysms approximate more to the forms of Belladonna or Drosera, with longer intervals. We might say, that in Veratrum the spasmodic element prevails; in Ipecacuanha the catarrhal one; thus the frequently decisive action of Veratrum in influenza, in simple spasmodic cough, in whooping cough, next to Belladonna, Drosera,

Conium, Cuprum, in nervous bronchial asthma, in stenosis of the glottis, or in angina pectoris."

Aggravations, coming from cold into a warm atmosphere; growing warm in bed; change of weather; damp, cold weather; eating and drinking cold things, as water, ice cream, &c.; morning and late in the evening.

PRACTICAL EXPEDIENTS

DEMULCENT BEVERAGES, of Barley water, Gum water, Rice water, or Toast water often of much service. They should be prepared as follows:—

Barley Water—One tablespoonful of pearl barley washed clean in cold water; then pour off the water and add the rind of one lemon, the juice of half a lemon, one teaspoonful of sugar; pour on one quart of boiling water, cover the vessel and let it stand for two hours; then strain. If the patient desires, the lemon can be omitted, and sliced liquorice, orange juice or currant jelly used instead.

Gum Water—Dissolve one ounce of clean gum-arabic, one half ounce of white sugar, in one pint of hot water. If desired the juice of lemon or orange can be added for flavoring. This is often very soothing to the cough.

Linseed Tea—Take one ounce of bruised linseed; half ounce of sliced liquorice root, to two pints of boiling water; macerate in a covered vessel before the fire, for three hours, then strain through a piece of muslin. This is a very soothing beverage in hard, teasing coughs. Dose, one tablespoonful as often as necessary. Lemon or orange juice will make it more palatable.

Rice Water—Wash the best rice with cold water, then boil in clean water for ten minutes, then the water should be strained off and more added, and so on till the goodness is all boiled out of the rice. When cold, the water is ready to drink; a little cream may be added, or some kind of flavoring if desired.

Toast Water—Take a crust of stale bread; bake slowly, not burn it; put it in a quart of boiling water; when cool, it is ready for use. This may be flavored with lemon peel.

Sulphurous Acid Spray has been found eminently beneficial in many cases of cough.

The London *Lancet* recommends a new remedy for cough: "Resistance to the desire to cough until the phlegm has accumulated in large quantities, when there will be something to cough against, and the phlegm may be brought up with much less effort. A great deal of the hacking, hemming and coughing in invalids in purely nervous, or the effect of habit, and exercise of the will is needed to prevent the wasteful exercise of power in cleaning the throat. Experiments in hospitals have shown this to be true."

Tar Water or capsules, taken three or six times a day as a common drink, not only acts as a palliative, but has cured hundreds of patients suffering with acute and chronic bronchitis. Acts better when the cough is moist.

WATER—In dry cough and bronchitis sicca, the inhalation of steam produces great relief; it restores the arrested circulation by stimulating the capillaries to contraction. Also, small quantities of cold water drunk at short intervals gives much temporary relief.

An excellent palliative in hard, dry, racking cough, is *dilute glycerine,* either with wine or whiskey.

Dr. Brown Sequard states that nervous cough may be checked by pressure on the nerves of the lip in the neighborhood of the nose, or in front of and near the ear, or very hard pressure on the top of the mouth inside, or by the strong exercise of will.

Rosin— In loose bronchial coughs we have used inhalation of the fumes of burning rosin, with pleasing effects. A small quantity of fine rosin is put into an old tea pot and set on fire with a few burning coals, and the vessel is set upon the patient's lap, when the fumes can be inhaled with great ease. Or it can be burned in a closed room. I like the tea pot the best, for pure air can be given to the patient constantly, which cannot be done in a small, closed room.

Cavities in the Lungs— A peculiar method of treating pulmonary cavities in phthisis, pursued by Prof. Mosler, of Wiesbaden, is described as consisting in the injection of certain drugs through the wall of the chest, and leaving the canula in, so as to repeat the operation at discretion. He has even made an incision into the walls of the cavity, inserted a silver tube or elastic catheter, and succeeded in drawing away the secretion and in disinfecting the pyogenic walls by means of a weak carbolic acid lotion. It is stated that no difficulty was experienced in the operation, and the condition of the patient was improved, the cough becoming less troublesome, and the febrile symptoms apparently moderated. One point, at least, is regarded as settled—and it is certainly of great importance—so far as could be by a few experiments of this character, namely, that the local treatment of pulmonary cavities is undoubtedly practicable, and that the lung is really more tolerant of external interference than has been generally believed."—*American Journal of Homœopahic Materia Medica,* Vol. iii. *page* 414.

ASTHMA

This is a constitutional affection, consisting of the spasmodic narrowing of the bronchial tubes, from contraction of the circular muscular fibres, with difficult expiration, great wheezing and a dreadful sense of constriction in the chest. In the majority of cases, it is the expression of perverted nervous action (neurosis), but not always a purely nervous disease. There are often organic diseases of the lungs, heart, brain or medulla oblongata, which produce the most obstinate cases of asthma, especially tuberculosis of the lungs.

We believe the cryptogamic theory of hay fever to be a fantasy. This autumnal catarrh is a constitutional affection, and no one can become affected by it, excepting those having this peculiar constitutional dyscrasia, and it requires no different treatment from common asthma.

TREATMENT

This is one of the most difficult and trying diseases the physician is called upon to treat. Not withstanding homoeopathy can boast of some brilliant cures of this disease, medical treatment is often unsatisfactory and uncertain.

Remedies for the Acute Attack—The most valuable and first to be studied are Ipecac, Veratrum viride, Digitaline,

ASTHMA

Arsenicum and Stramonium. Second: such remedies as Aconite, Acid hydrocyanicum, Ambra, Belladonna, Bryonia, Chamomilla, Coffea, Cannabis sativa, China, Camphora, Gelsemium, Hyoscyamus, Lobelia, Lachesis, Morphine, Opium, Musk, Nux vomica, Pulsatilla, Sanguinaria, Sabadilla, Tartar emetic, Tobacco and Veratrum album.

CHRONIC ASTHMA—The most useful remedies are, Arsenicum, Calcarea carb., Cod liver oil, Ferrum, Glanderine, Iodium, Kali i, Lycopodium, Mercury and Sulphur. Second: such remedies as Argentum nitricum, Aurum, Ammonium carb., Bromine, Causticum, Carbo veg., Graphites, Hepar sulphuris Kali nit., Kali bi., Kali br., Mercury, Nitric acid, Natrium m., Phosphorus, Spongia, Sepia, Stannum and Zinc.

We will now give the leading indications of the most valuable of the above mentioned remedies in an alphabetical order. In this way we hope to be able to cover all kinds and cases of asthma.

ACONITUM NAPELLUS—Great fear and anxiety of mind, with nervous excitability; high fever, full bounding pulse and agonized tossing about; great fear of death; sure he will die; vertigo on sitting up in bed; asthma brought on from change of temperature from warm to intensely cold weather; dry cough. Sanguine, plethoric people, who are very irritable and sensitive; symptoms greatly aggravated at night, especially after midnight.

This remedy is more especially useful to a subdue the acute attack. It's sphere of usefulness is soon passed. Cases that Aconite is adapted to are young plethoric people, with cerebral hyperemia, accompanied with intense fear; *congestive nervous* asthma. Dr. E.H. Ruddock says: "The striking power of this pneumogastric nerve, characterized by imperfect and labored breathing, has suggested it's use in *spasmodic asthma,* during the *paroxysms* of which we have often administered it with marked and speedy relief. It is especially indicated by oppressive anxiety, dyspnea, and labored action of the heart. It is the best palliative in bronchitic asthma.

Dr. T. Nichol says: "For the last fifteen years the writer has been in the habit of looking upon *Aconite* as one of the very chief of our anti-spasmodic remedies, and of late years the same view has been taken by some of our best writers." Hempel asserts that in "spasmodic asthma, when resulting from exposure to keen wind, or from the retrocession of some acute eruption, acute nettle rash, or the like, *Aconite* will be found invaluable; the orthopnea of Aconite is equivalent to an attack of spasmodic asthma."

Dr. Hughes says: "When the asthma is bronchitic, I agree with Drs. Russell and Blandell in considering Aconite the best palliative. It might have been added, that the remedy is curative as well as palliative. Aconite, then, is the appropriate remedy when the patient is of full plethoric habits, when the asthma is from a sudden cold; also in cases in which the attack follows the suppression of an acute rash. Oppressive anxiety, dyspnea and labored action of the heart are leading indications, and unless these are present, but little good need be expected from it. The cough often comes on at night, and is rough, spasmodic, croaking, as if the patient would suffocate, with hoarse, barking voice, and spasmodic constriction of the chest and throat; respiration is short, anxious and difficult, with an open mouth and an inability to utter a single word distinctly. There seems to be a constriction of the chest present, and as the spasm relaxes, the expectoration is yellowish or blood streaked. During the attack, the patient is peevish, restless and irritable, and even in young children the characteristic dread of death is seen. The pulse is small, irregular and intermittent, and the heat of the surface is considerable. All dilutions have cured, but I prefer the triturations from the 4th to the 12th given in repeated doses."

ARSENICUM ALBUM—Rapid and great prostration, with sinking of the vital forces; burning pains; the parts burn like fire; intense thirst; drinks little, and often; craves warm air; great anguish, restlessness, and fear of death; excessive restlessness, cannot lie still; relieved by motion; great emaciation; cannot lie down for fear of suffocation; highest degree of dyspnea; sad and irritable; anasarca of the whole body; obstinate nausea and vomiting; cadaverous diarrhea, with great enervation; cold night sweats.

For chronic organic cases Arsenicum is one of the most useful remedies we have for this trying disease. My friend, Dr. T. Nichol, has given such a practical *résumé* of it's action in his article on "The Respiratory Affections of Childhood," that I cannot do better than give it in full. He says: "Opinions differ very much as to the value of Arsenicum in asthma. Dr. Bags, whose bright book is one of the most readable that has appeared of late years, says that 'in asthma I have seen occasional good results from Arsenicum, but have never seen it cured by this medicine'; while Dr. B. Baehr, whose great work entitles him to rank as an authority of the first class, avers that 'Arsenicum is undoubtedly the safest remedy for asthma. It not only corresponds to the secondary forms of asthma, which owe their existence to the most diversified affections of a more primary character.' Kreussler asserts that, 'in cases of years' standing, Arsenic affords only temporary relief, although it is perfectly adapted to the severest of recent asthma'; while Ruddock, at least of equal value as an authority, says 'that it is especially useful in chronic asthma;' and Dr. Hughes says that 'Arsenicum is the best medicine where bronchitic asthma tends to become, or has become, chronic.' Dr. Laurie considers that in confirmed asthmatics, it forms a most important remedy. In my own practice I have repeatedly seen radical cures of both acute and chronic asthma with this remedy, though I agree with Dr. Ruddock that it is of especial value in the chronic form."

Arsenicum is an invaluable remedy when the asthma results from suppressed eruptions, and when it also attacks children of feeble and impaired constitutions. It is also of great service when the asthma—which is here merely symptomatic, not idiopathic—depends on disease of the heart, or upon pulmonary emphysema or œdema, or upon chronic bronchitis. Dr. Nuñez, of Madrid, affirms that Arsenicum is curative in the nervous asthma, resulting from the suppression of dry eruptions, such as lichen on the palm of the hand. All experienced practitioners can confirm Baehr's remark, that, "in the asthmatic paroxysms of tuberculous patients, Arsenic has always left us in the lurch."

Baehr says: "We dispense with the enumeration of individual symptoms, since every somewhat violent attack of asthma corresponds to arsenic." Baehr is one of the first minds in our school, and he has perhaps no greater admirer on this side of the Atlantic than the writer, but I most emphatically dissent from a statement which strikes at that individualization of cases which is the essence of homœopathy. Is Arsenicum adapted to *all* cases of asthma, without exception? Surely not. If not, then *we must diagnose the remedy as well as the disease.*

"The Arsenicum asthma, as a general rule, attacks fiercely and soon reaches it's acme. The more the patients seem on the point of suffocating, the more painful and distressing the restlessness; the more wheezing and louder the respirations, the more Arsenicum will be found appropriate."—*Baehr.*

Laurie remarks that this remedy is indicated when the paroxysms of asthma are most liable to occur when retiring to rest, or before midnight, the patient being disturbed from sleep by a sense of spasmodic constriction in the chest and upper part of the windpipe, which is soon followed by laborious panting and whistling respiration, with gasping for breath.

ASTHMA

The respiration is attended with extreme agitation, restlessness and moaning; extreme anguish and exhaustion, as if at the point of death, with cold perspiration. The dyspnea is difficult and stifling, with suffocative attacks, recurring in paroxysms. The cough is frequent, dry, and exhaustive, and is attended with constriction in the trachea, and followed by suffocative fits. There is often an accumulation of thick phlegm, and the paroxysms grow lighter on the appearance of cough with expectoration of mucus or viscid saliva. There are also violent palpitations of the heart present, with a small, quick and intermittent pulse, together with dry, burning heat, alternating with cold perspiration. The prostration is extreme, and children who are old enough complain of the well known burning heat in the chest. The face is pale or bluish, with an anxious or desponding expression. The consequences of the paroxysm remain for a long time, and prostration and nervous debility are peculiarly prominent.

The asthmatic paroxysm to which Arsenicum corresponds is excited by active exertion, even by getting into bed; by talking or laughing; by changes in the atmospheric temperature, and also by warm or tight clothing. The paroxysm is aggravated by lying down, and relieved by sitting erect and by bending forward; to which Hartmann adds, that "the patient cannot speak a word without making the asthma worse."

Arsenicum is well known to be adapted to night paroxysms, but it is likewise suitable to attacks coming on during the day.

As to the dose, Marcy says that "the first to the third trituration may be employed regulating the repetition according to the urgency of the symptoms." Drs. Marcy and Hunt give still larger doses, and advise the exhibition of a preparation of Arsenic seldom used in Homœopathic practice, "the Liquor Arsenicalis, which is said to be much more efficacious than

Arsenicum album seems to be prompt and energetic when Arsenicum is indicated. It should be prepared with distilled water instead of alcohol. The most efficacious and satisfactory method of treating asthma is with the Arsenical solution—1st dilution, and Kali i, first decimal trituration, in alternation, every hour or two, or three times a day, as circumstances demand. Baehr judiciously remarks : "During the apyrexia the remedy had better be administered at long intervals and in the higher attenuations, although the success which 'old school' practitioners have attained with Fowler's solution, justifies the conclusion that massive doses are likewise conducive to a cure. The danger is that massive doses may affect the stomach injuriously. My own experience is in favor of the administration from the 12th trituration to the 30th dilution during the interval, giving the 6th to the 12th decimal trituration, during and immediately after the actual attack. I have had no experience with Fowler's solution."

My experience with Fowler's solution has been so favorable that I do not hesitate to state, that it is twice as useful as Arsenicum album I use the first three attenuations (decimal scale), and sometimes the pure solution in drop doses. Twice I have given the $1,000^{th}$ (Tafel's) attenuation of Arsenicum album, with immediate and lasting curative results.

AURUM METALLICUM—Great melancholy; the mind constantly tends towards self destruction; utter despair; swelling, and exostosis of the skull bones; nightly bone pains; syphilitico-mercurial affections; oversensitiveness to pain and cold air; indurated glands; worse in warm air and wet weather.

Chronic organic cases, with perfect despair and loathing of life. "Where it is not certain whether the heart is primarily or secondarily involved in the attack, the attack sets in with violent palpitations of the heart, great anxiety and marked symptoms of pulmonary hyperemia.

AMMONIUM CARBONICUM—Weak, nervous people, or lymphatic, venous temperaments. The moment he falls asleep he is aroused again for want of breath; great hæmorrhages; scurvy; worse evenings and during wet weather; anasarca; hydrothorax; bronchorrhea.

Organic cases. Hartmann says: "Asthma with repeated palpitations of the heart, considerable œdema of the feet, and an asthmatic state every evening, continuing until midnight, relieved by the open air; dyspnea with palpitations of the heart when moving; heaviness and burning in the chest, aggravated in wet weather, relieved by warmth and dry weather.

ARGENTUM NITRICUM—Time passes too slow; everything done seems to be done too slow; excessive flatulence; stomach nearly ready to burst with gas; fluid seems to run straight through the intestinal canal without stopping; diarrhea from ulceration of the intestines.

Severe organic cases that are much worse at night. The attacks commence suddenly, with very distressing shortness of breath; tension as if a band was around the præcordia; very short breath, with deep sighs, and violent palpitations of the heart, or oppressed panting, quick, sibilant breathing, inability to lie down, obliged to lean forward to get breath, with rumbling of gas in the chest and bowels.

From the first to the third decimal will be found of great utility.

AMBRA GRISEA—Hysterical, nervous females; spasmodic, choking sensation in the throat, with frequent fainting fits; dry spasmodic cough; aggravated in the evening; relieved in the open air; loud eructations of gas.

Asthma in nervous, hysterical women. As a palliative Ambra is of great use, Hartmann says: "I have found *Ambra,* second or third trituration, an useful remedy in asthma siccum and senile, particularly when the oppression was principally felt in the left chest, extending from the heart to the back and between the shoulders, attended with palpitations, anguish, arrest of breathing. It likewise proved useful in asthmatic ailments of scrofulous subjects."

Greatly aggravated at night and in a warm atmosphere.

Amber beads worn about the neck have a wonderful reputation of curing hay fever.

> **ACIDUM HYDROCYAUM**—Spasms of the face and muscles of the back, and the body assumes a bluish tint. Long fainting spells, violent palpitations of the heart; paralysis of the oesophagus, the fluid runs gurgling down the oesophagus; much rattling of mucus, with sluggish respiration.

This remedy has a most powerful action upon the medulla oblongata and spinal cord, and ought to be one of our main remedies in spasmodic asthma. "Professor Geise had suffered for a long time, both day and night, with periodical asthma, and the most violent attacks of suffocative spasmodic cough, which had withstood all remedies. Acidum hydrocynicum, two drops per dose, three times a day, cured in five weeks.

"A middle aged man, who had repeatedly suffered from profuse spitting of blood, finally became permanently asthmatic. As the disease progressed, it became more and more spasmodic, and to a certain degree periodical, although organic disease of the chest was suspected. Twelve days' treatment with Acidum hydrocynicum entirely cured the case, after a fruitless use of several remedies, internal and external."—*Frank.*

> **BELLADONNA**—Pains come and go with great celerity; furious delirium, wild look, wishes to strike, bite or quarrel; face flushed; eyes red; rage, tears, bites and strikes; violent throbbing of the carotids; throbbing headache; worse by motion; noise is intolerable; great dryness of the fauces; bright, red and swollen tonsils; spasms of the throat; symptoms worse evenings and at night.

As a palliative, in acute cases, Bell. is frequently of great value. Baehr says : "When the attack is accompanied by congestion of the head and an affection of the larynx in the case of plethoric individuals, children and females of an irritable disposition."

Bell. has been especially recommended in cases occurring in females of an irritable constitution, also in cases where there exists a tendency to spasm, or any organic lesion.

Hartmann asserts that it "often proves radically curative after the exhibition of some intercurrent remedy, particularly in cases which have not become too chronic by repeated relapses, under which circumstances we must take recourse in Sulphur, Calc. or some other antipsoric."

It is particularly called for when the paroxysms come on in fits of short, difficult, irregular and suffocating respiration, accompanied by dry cough; pressure on the chest, violent beating of the heart, vertigo, swimming or darting pains in the head, pains in the small of the back and limbs, cramps in different parts of the body, anxiety, irritability and fretfulness." *Marcy and Hunt.*

These symptoms are greatly aggravated in the evening and at night. Atropine sometimes acts better than Belladonna.

> **BRYONIA ALBA**—All the symptoms are greatly aggravated by motion; dry cough, compels the patient to sit up immediately; respiration oppressed; wishes to take in a long breath but cannot; feeling as if the lungs could not expand; constipation; dry, hard, burnt looking stools; lips parched, dry and cracked; worse nights and from warmth; severe stiching pains during inspiration.

Dr. Nichol says : "Bryonia is the appropriate remedy where the asthma originates from, or is complicated with catarrhal and pulmonary maladies, and it is of use in cases arising from suppressed eruptions or partially developed rashes. The leading symptoms of the Bryonia asthma is, that it is worse by motion, and at night, with pain in the chest.

The paroxysms of Bryonia asthma usually occur at night, and it is almost invariably preceded by catarrhal symptoms, difficult breathing and loss of breath, especially at night and toward morning, aggravation of dyspnea from talking or from the slightest movement. This difficulty in breathing is often accompanied by stitching pains, inability to lie on the right side, and not without inconvenience on the left, so that the patient is constrained to lie on the back; frequent efforts to obtain sufficient air by deep inspiration, accompanied with moaning palpitations of the heart, and great anxiety. The cough is hard and frequent, with expectoration at first frothy and subsequently thick and glutinous, frequently attended with retching and vomiting; the patient feels relieved after expectorating, or rising from a recumbent position; frequent stitches in the chest, especially during an inspiration, and when coughing, also during motion; at other times there are oppressive, tensive or contractive pains in the chest, and the asthmatic attacks are often attended by shootings in the lungs on taking a full inspiration, also on coughing or after any movement of the arms or trunk. Often gastric symptoms are present, bitter or acid eructations, or eructations tasting of the food, colic, pressive pains in the head increased by motion, and the characteristic mental symptoms prevail; irritability of temper and a disposition to find fault with everything.

Laurie and Caspari say that Bryonia and Nux v. are often administered with great advantage in alternation, and Ruff reports a cure which followed these remedies given in that manner. But as the symptoms of Bryonia are quite distinct from those of Nux v., it will be better and more scientific practice to discriminate carefully between them, and then give the indicated remedy singly and alone. More valuable is Jahr's therapeutic hint, that Bryonia is frequently suitable after Ipecac in acute asthma.

BROMIUM—Suffocating cough, with hoarse wheezing and gasping, with a false membrane in the trachea, especially where the larynx and trachea are inflamed; great rattling of mucus in the larynx and trachea when coughing; great nervous prostration, remaining after all other symptoms have gone; aggravation in the evening.

In organic cases, where there is a great collection of mucus in the trachea and lungs, second stage of asthma. Dr. Douglas says : "A dyspnea of ten years standing, in a girl sixteen years of age, which had remained after measles, and was so violent that the girl was sometimes not able to walk fast or go up stairs without feeling very much exhausted, disappeared after taking five doses of Bromine 30, five pellets each. It is one of the few drugs that produce the croupous false membrane in the air passages."

Wheezing, rattling breathing, with a tight feeling in the chest, accompanied with a dry, spasmodic, wheezing cough, worse in the forepart of the night and in a warm room.

> **CALCAREA CARBONICA**—Leuco-phlegmatic constitutions; large head and features, pale, flabby skin, with chalky looks, and in infants open fontanelles; profuse perspiration on the head, stands out in large, bead like drops, often soaks the pillow thoroughly; much peevishness; food is badly assimilated; great debility; in going up stairs is out of breath, has to sit down; running up stairs produces great vertigo; feet feel cold continually, as if he had on cold, damp stockings; acid stomach with sour vomiting; swelling over the pit of the stomach like a saucer turned bottom upward; chronic watery diarrhea. In women the menses are too often, too profuse and last too long; loose, rattling cough; great emaciation, the least cold goes through and through the patient; hectic fever, with copious perspiration on the head and chest; cold, damp, east wind is sure to bring on a cold.

Calcarea is one of the most useful and reliable remedies we have to eradicate the constitutional dyscrasia that lies at the foundation of asthma, and should be thoroughly studied in all cases of chronic, organic cases of asthma, especially if the person afflicted is a child. Calc. has a marvellous effect upon children that are growing rapidly, and are afflicted with asthma. Also affects the female organism more favorably than that of a man. Acts best in leuco-phlegmatic, scrofulous constitutions, where the organic or ganglionic nervous system is at fault, as shown by great emaciation and debility. The asthmatic breathing is accompanied with a feeling of tightness in the chest as if too full of blood and loud mucous rales, with soreness in the chest when drawing a deep breath and touching it; the cough sounds loose, but little is expectorated. There is often a sensation as if there was dust in the throat and lungs; attack comes on early in the morning; it is almost impossible for the patient to go up stairs, or to ascend any height. It is the peculiar scrofulous dyscrasia that Calcarea is adapted to, rather than particular symptoms. Dr. G. V. Miller says of *Calcarea phosphorica:*—"Subjects instead of being

ASTHMA

fat, as in *Calc. carb.* are emaciated. Instead of a clear, white complexion like the above, it is for a dirty white or brown complexion; also, skull is soft, thin, crepitating when pressed, especially on the occiput. Craves bacon, salt meat and potatoes."

> **CANNABIS SATIVA**—Acute cases, where the mucous membrane of the lungs is loaded with mucus; sensation as if cold water were dropping over the heart or head; bloody urine; sexual over excitement; humid asthma.

In the second or sub-acute stage of humid asthma. "Humid asthma, extreme agitation, dyspnea, wheezing and mucous rales. As the attack declines, an easy rattling cough brings up copious, thick, yellow sputa."—*Ruddock.*

"When the patient can only breathe in a sitting posture with the neck stretched forward, wheezing in the trachea; abdominal muscles put violently on the stretch during every inspiration, exceedingly restless and tortured by anguish. These symptoms occurred before midnight, in a patient suffering with organic heart disease, and the effect of Cannabis was very striking."—*Hartmann.*

> **CAUSTICUM**—Scrofulous people, with yellow complexion; cannot keep the upper eyelids open, they will fall down over the eyes; great melancholy, looks on the dark side of everything, especially so in women during menstruation; acid stomach, with much flatulence; obstinate constipation; painful pustules near the anus, discharging pus, blood and serum; no remedy has so many anal symptoms; involuntary urination when coughing; chronic morning hoarseness; *complete aphonia;* wheezing cough, the expectoration cannot be spit out, is obliged to swallow what is raised. Worse in cold, dry weather.

This is a ganglionic remedy of penetrating action, and is especially useful in old organic chronic cases, to eradicate that peculiar asthmatic dyscrasia. Not so useful as a palliative, but of much value as a constitutional remedy.

"Asthma when sitting or lying down; tight dressing oppresses breathing; dry, wheezing, whistling, hoarse, hollow cough, with soreness in the chest; expectoration only at night, which he cannot raise, but has to swallow it again; involuntary passage of urine when coughing, aggravated by cold air and in the evening." In cases adapted to Caust. there is much hoarseness, loss of voice, and an excessively dark yellow complexion.

> **CARBO VEGETABILIS**—Weak, cachectic people, with great foulness of the secretions, especially the sputa; craves more air, wants to be fanned all the time; spongy gums that bleed readily; excessive accumulation of gas in the stomach and bowels, with a sensation as if the stomach or abdomen would burst; constant eructations of flatus, by the mouth and anus; slimy diarrhea; icy coldness of the parts; tendency to gangrene; much hoarseness; very offensive breath and sputa.

This remedy is useful in the second stage of chronic organic cases, where there is great wheezing and much rattling of mucus in the lungs, and expectoration is abundant in the morning. "Much oppression of breathing, with wheezing; rattling mucus, and a hoarse, loose cough, more especially in the morning. Cough, with spitting of blood or pus, with marked burning distress in the lungs." Aggravated in cold, damp, wet weather and cold air.

> **CHAMOMILLA**—Especially acts upon the sensory and excito-motor systems. Out of humor, very impatient, cannot answer one civilly, the pains make him furious, the least thing makes him fretful; asthma brought on by a fit of passion; in children, one cheek red and the other pale; tongue coated yellow; flatulent colic. Diarrhea green and watery, or like chopped eggs. Dry, hacking cough, worse in the open air and at night.

In the peculiar temperament that calls for Chamomilla, this remedy will be found valuable in nervous, spasmodic asthma, especially if the "attack is caused by a severe fit of passion, with flatulence, particularly for a paroxysm of hysteric asthma, or for children during dentition."—*Baker.*

"Chamomilla is an important remedy in the flatulent asthma of children, also in that following a suppressed catarrh. It is likewise, specific in attacks which are caused by anger, grief, fear, &c., in adults. Distention and sensation of fullness in the stomach and bowels; pressure, anxiety, and fulness in the region of the heart; short wheezing respiration; great restlessness; dry irritating cough; bad taste; tainted breath."—*Marcy & Hunt.*

> **CHINA**—The system has been debilitated by the loss of vital fluids, especially blood, semen, over lactation, diarrhea, or leucorrhea. Patient worse every other day. Intermittant neuralgia, greatly aggravated by the slightest touch. Much congestion of blood to the head, with ringing in the ears. Loss of appetite, with longing for acids. Dirty yellow coating upon the tongue. Acid stomach, with much flatulence. Abdomen seems packed full of gas, not relieved by eructations or dejections. Diarrhea, of undigested food or water, without pain. Jaundice. Dark, scanty urine. Metrorrhagia and menorrhagia. Debilitating night sweats. Intermittent congestion of the lungs.

This is not a true asthmatic remedy, but may be a valuable one in cases that assume an intermittent type, in debilitated, cachectic subjects, living in a malarious atmosphere. The digestive organs are in a debilitated condition as is shown by excessive flatulence; the abdomen is distended with gas like a drum; there is diarrhea and excessive debility. Pale, sallow countenance; the paroxysms come on worse after midnight, and in wet weather; the patient has exhausting night sweats especially affecting the chest. Oppression of the chest from excessive flatulence. Suffocative fits, as from mucus in the larynx. Symptoms aggravated by a draft of air or the slightest contact.

CAMPHORA OFFICINALIS—Sudden prostration of the vital forces, with excessive coldness of the external surface. Long lasting chills. Skin cold as marble, yet cannot bear to be covered. Extremities cold and blue, with cramps. First stages of catarrhal affections. Involuntary diarrhea. Retention of urine. Humid asthma.

For the first stage of suffocative asthma, where there seems danger of paralysis of the vagi, Camphor is of great value; but it's stage of usefulness is soon passed, and we must find another remedy.

Hartmann says: "Camphor is likewise a palliative, but only in certain cases. I use it in asthma humidum with very irritable nerves, and particularly when the larynx and bronchial tubes are so filled with mucus that the patient is almost suffocated, which is easily inferred by the movement of the patient's hands and by the spasmodic contortion of the facial muscles."

In the so called "hay asthma," Dr. Holcomb has used the 1st centesimal trituration with marked effect.

COD LIVER OIL— For asthma, in young, growing children, to eradicate that peculiar dyscrasia, that lays the foundation of asthma, we have no better remedy than Cod liver oil, and no long standing, organic case ought to be treated without it's use. I have seen good results from it's use, but believe, however, that it is more useful in young people than in the aged. I have derived great benefit from the oil in chronic, humid coughs of old people when other remedies have entirely failed. For it's action and use the reader is referred to the first part of this work.

CUPRUM METALLICUM—Sudden paroxysms of dyspnea. Strong metallic taste in the mouth. Spasmodic affections generally. Sudden, severe vomiting. When drinking, the fluid descends with a gurgling noise. Chlorotic symptoms. Chronic asthma.

ASTHMA

The main sphere of Cuprum is to eradicate the tendency to asthma; is not of much value to relieve the paroxysms.

"The remedy is suitable to individuals with nervous, irritable, enfeebled constitutions, who are more over, disposed to spasms, where as Arsenicum is suitable to rather vigorous and plethoric persons. Or it is suitable to children, especially if the spasms set in at night, or in consequence of exerting the respiratory organs, as for instance, after a coughing fit; the paroxysm very speedily reaches the acme of it's intensity; other muscular bundles are involved in the convulsive attack; the attack is accompanied by a constant hacking, which aggravates the asthma, and it terminates by vomiting; pallor of the countenance, with cold perspiration. The apyrexia is not perfect, but a light degree of dyspnea remains, or violent paroxysms of an almost dry cough set in, which likewise end in vomiting. We have never known Cuprum to be of any use for the paroxysm itself, so that we now limit the use of this drug exclusively to the intervals between the paroxysms."—*Baehr.*

"Cough; painful contraction of the chest; losing of breath; great weakness and relaxation of body; emaciation; loss of spirits; anxiety, fits of anguish and fear of death; when trying to take a deep breath, cough with whistling breathing; dyspnea in spasmodic fits, almost suffocating; aggravation at night, also when coughing, when leaning backwards and after drinking." —*Dr. H. Goullon.*

> DIGITALINE—The great keynote this remedy is an intermittent pulse, or where the least movement produces violent palpitations of the heart; dropsy of the pericardium, in organic heart diseases; feeling of goneness in the stomach, as if he would die with deathly nausea and vomiting; white or ash coloured stools; spermatorrhea; bloating and paleness of the face; anasarca;

> humid asthma, with great rattling of mucus in the lungs; cyanosis and fainting. Paroxysms come on early in the morning, and in cold weather.

This remedy, in all probability if the active principle *Digitaline* is given, has no superior in our *materia medica*, not only to relieve the paroxysms, but also to radically cure the disease. I no more use the *Digitalis*, it being not more than half as useful as the alkaloid, Digitaline, and always use it in the second or third centesimal trituration. This, I regret to state, was omitted in my "Characteristic Materia Medica," and has been the cause of several communications in our journals. I hope physicians will make a note of this.

Dr. B. Baehr says: "In a variety of cases we have witnessed remarkably favorable results from the use Digitaline. With this remedy alone we have radically cured frequently recurring paroxysms of asthma of a less protracted duration; in inveterate cases all that we have been able to accomplish with this agent, has been to diminish, in some cases, although to a considerable extent, the intensity and frequency of the paroxysm; it is, therefore, with a good conscience that we can recommend this medicine for further trails in asthma, provided the following circumstances are kept in view : asthma is altogether a primary affection; it is the purely nervous in form, a genuine spasm of the bronchi. In such a case Digitaline will have the best effect as long as no catarrh, emphysema or structural change of the heart supervenes. Digitaline is, however, suitable even if these complications exist, to which it is, indeed, preëminently adapted, more especially to structural alterations of the right ventricle. A high degree of sanguinous stasis in the veins of the head, especially a violent throbbing, pressing headache during and after the attack; palpitations of the heart, especially if the attack is preceded by them. The asthma attacks irritable individuals with weak nerves, more particularly persons who

ASTHMA

have been guilty of sexual excesses. We do not simply mean persons who have been addicted to self abuse, for we have known a married man who contracted asthmatic attacks in consequence of excessive sexual intercourse, and who was decidedly benefitted by Digitaline. The influence of Digitaline over the male sexual organs is extraordinary, and in this case, we effected a truly radical cure, as is like wise evident from what we stated when speaking of the male sexual organs, especially in it's bearing upon the nervous system, is so difficult to define that we are as yet without any decided data regarding this matter. We always administer this remedy in the second or third trituration, giving never more than one grain of the former in the morning before breakfast, never at night, for the reason that sleep is generally disturbed by Digitaline. (I cannot subscribe to this. I am in the habit of repeating it every two or three hours, and it greatly quietens the patient instead of producing restlessness). Nor is it necessary to give a dose every day; a dose every two or three days is sufficient. These precautions are important to avoid medicinal effects and homœopathic aggravations. Unless these precautionary measures are adopted, a remedy, the great importance of which has not yet been sufficiently recognized, might easily fall into discredit."

Hartmann says: "This medicine is useful in asthma complicated with thoracic disorganization. It is supposed that Digitalis is indicated by a disturbed action of the heart and slow pulse; but I have always employed it with success when the disturbed action of the heart manifested itself equally in the pulse. The increased action of the heart depended upon incipient disorganization of that organ and it's vessels, and the asthma caused by that disorganization was characterized by the following symptoms : roughness in the trachea, which had existed for some time previous, accompanied with a short, hacking cough, and gradually leading to labored breathing, which increases to a spasmodic constriction of the larynx and chest, with suffocative anguish, which is particularly troublesome early in the morning, on waking and obliges one to sit up. Digitalis is, therefore, an excellent remedy for asthma cardicum, organicum, metastaticum and hydrothoracicum." "Digitalis is indicated in those cases where the respiration is slow, pulse is slow or intermitting the third, fifth, or seventh beat; face of a bluish red colour; sweat on upper part of the body and tendency to diarrhea. The paroxysms come on early in the morning, especially in cold weather." —RAUE.

> **FERRUM METALLICUM**—Weak, chlorotic, anæmic people. The least emotion, or exertion, produces a red, flushed face; very pale, anæmic people, the least motion produces a bright, red face; great paleness of the mucous membranes, especially that of the cavity of the mouth; muscles feeble and easily exhausted from slight exertion. Always better from walking about slowly, not withstanding weakness obliges the patient to lie down; acid, sour vomiting, lienteria, obstinate, painless diarrhea, excoriating and exhausting. In women, menses too frequent, too profuse and last too long; watery leucorrhea; hæmoptysis and a general hæmorrhagic tendency; rheumatism of the deltoid muscle; general anasarca; cold extremities.

In cachectic leucophlegmatic individuals, where there is great anæmia and the blood making organs are completely prostrated, Ferrum will be found the main remedy in our hands to build up again the debilitated organism. It does this by entering the circulation, and there it stimulates the organic nerves which preside over the blood making organs until sanguinous process goes on in a normal manner. Iron is not a remedy with which to arrest the paroxysm of asthma, but will be of great value to build up the worn out organism between the paroxysms. If the attack comes on after midnight, driving the patient out of bed, and is relieved by walking about slowly, iron will be strongly indicated. Also, if there is great congestion of blood to the head, with puffiness around the eyes; throbbing headache; vertigo and roaring in the head; walking produces faintness; anxiety and oppression proceeding from the pit of the stomach; tightness in the chest, as if constricted; diffcult and anxious breathing, most violent when lying or sitting still, relieved by walking slowly or talking.

"A child, aged one year and a half, suffered with repeated attacks of Kopp's asthma, so that he often became unconscious. His digestion was good, but his muscles weak, so that he could not stand or walk; fontanelles were unusually large. Cured by Ferrum sulphuricum, internally and in baths."
—FRANK.

Anæmia and debility are the great signals for the use of iron, especially if there is a tendency of congestion of blood to the chest, emaciation and cold extremities.

> **GELSEMIUM SEMPERVIRENS**—Nervous, hysterical females and onanists, intense congestion of blood to the head; great heaviness of the eye lids; amaurosis; spermatorrhea, with great languor and irritability; hysterical spasms; nervous asthma, with profound prostration of the whole muscular system; constant sneezing.

This remedy is adapted to what might be called neurotic, hysterical asthma, the nervous or hysterical element predominating. It has a specific action on the nerves of the larynx and on Miller's asthma (laryngismus stridulus), it is one of our most useful and reliable remedies.

> **GRAPHITES**—Females inclined to obesity and a disposition to delayed menstruation, menses too late, pale and scanty; obstinate constipation; excessive flatulence; eruptions on the skin, oozing out a sticky fluid; acrid secretions, the skin becomes excoriated; every injury of the skin tends to suppurate; burning on top of the head and of the feet; great debility; suppressed eruptions.

This remedy is only useful to eradicate the peculiar dyscrasia lying at the foundation of asthma, in people prone to obesity, and in women there is a great tendency to delayed and scanty menstruation. The asthmatic paroxysm comes on in the evening; there is great sensitiveness to cold air and a liability to take cold at every change of weather.

"Suffocative paroxysms every night since 17 years in a man aged 70. The paroxysms awaken him from sleep, usually after midnight; he would quickly jump out of bed, and hold on to something, and quickly eat a piece of bread. After this the paroxysm passes off; and he can sleep. He had no other spell after Graphites 30 although he lived 8 years longer." Dr. Landesmann.

Glanderine—Dr. O. P. Baehr says that Glanderine is the true similimum, if it can be obtained pure. He does not give the indications for the kind of asthma, and never having used this remedy I cannot supply the want, but should judge that it might prove useful in the humid form, where there is much bronchial inflammation attended by profuse expectoration, accompanied with chronic catarrh.

> **HEPAR SULPHURIS**—Organic cases attended with suppuration and a rattling choking cough. Much hoarseness with laryngo-tracheal catarrh, cannot bear to be uncovered, cough when any part of the body is uncovered; constant tendency of the head and chest to perspire; sweats day and night without relief, especially about the chest; sour smelling perspiration; symptoms

worse during cold north-west winds, relieved by warmth; system has been abused by mercury; glandular swellings, especially of the tonsils. The skin is very sensitive to the slightest touch, even the clothes irritate him; great sensitiveness to everything; cannot bear the slightest draft of air, nor the slightest noise.

This is one of the most useful remedies we have in chronic cases of asthma, where the attack comes on in the night, with constriction of the chest and suffocative breathing; the patient has a *choking cough,* and a large collection of mucus in the bronchi. Tuberculosis or chronic bronchitis is at the foundation of the asthma.

"Hepar sulphuris must not be forgotten in those cases which awaken the patient from a sound sleep. During the paroxysm the face becomes blue, the saliva is increased and the patient complains of dust in the lungs; smoking (tobacco) and throwing the head back ameliorate; the expectoration after the attack is frothy." *Raue.*

Not of much value to relieve the paroxysms, but of great value to eradicate the peculiar dyscrasia, that lays at the foundation of asthma.

IPECACUANHA—Continuous and unavailable desire to vomit; constant nausea; no relief obtained by vomiting; great paleness of the face; the chest seems full of phlegm, but does not yield to coughing; suffocation threatens from constriction in the throat and chest; worse from the least motion; loses breath with the cough, turns pale in the face and stiffens; incessant sneezing large secretion of mucus in the nostrils.

To arrest the paroxysms of asthma, especially in little children, Ipecac is equal to any drug we have in the *materia medica.* Dr. T. Nichol has given us such a practical résmué of it's indications in asthma that I cannot serve the profession better than to give his remarks in full. He says: "Ipecacuanha is one of the first remedies of which we think of in an attack of acute asthma, and it is worthy of the place which it holds. It is a leading remedy in recent cases, particularly in young children, and it is likely to be indicated in cases caused by the suppression of miliaria or urticaria, and also by the inhalation of dust or irritating vapors. Dr. Hughes remarks : "It is in this variety (the bronchitic) that I consider Ipecac homœopathic, and not, as Dr. Russell seems to think, to pure nervous cases. It is especially indicated where there is much cough." Dr. Laurie says: "During a paroxysm of acute asthma, this remedy is one of the most frequently used, whether the attack occurs in children or adults." Almost the only unfavorable testimony the writer has seen is from Dr. Bayes, who, in the frank manner which gives such a peculiar charm to his writings, says: 'In asthma, Ipecac has disappointed me, I have seen some benefit from it's use, but far less than I was led to expect from it's pathogenesis." "The leading indications for this remedy are, spasmodic constriction of the air passages and accumulation of mucus in them; feeling of tightness in the chest, which may be quite distinctly made out even in very young children by stripping them and noting the motions of the chest, with rattling and panting in the windpipe which is full of mucus; the cough is short, dry and troublesome, with quick and laborious breathing, and a good deal of gasping for breath; sometimes the cough appears to be excited by a tickling commencing in the upper part of the throat and extending to the extreme ramifications of the bronchial tubes; at other times, the stethoscope shows that the spasmodic constriction of the bronchial tubes is the essence of the morbid state; nausea with cold sweat on the forehead is also present, with a small and slow pulse, or nausea before the attack and vomiting, mostly bile, during, or nausea before or after the attack; the tongue is coated and the appetite is deficient. The face is pale and cold, and

ASTHMA

this state sometimes alternates with heat and redness; the hands and feet are cold and in aggravated cases, there is tetanic rigidity of the body, with lividity or a bluish redness of the face; the mind is anxious and morose, or irritability, impatience and fear of death are present.

As to the dose, practitioners vary greatly. Caspari advises the third attenuation, either one drop in water, or in the form of globules, repeating it every two or three hours, as it's action is soon over; and Hale for all the remedies he mentions for this disease, directs a dose of three or four globules to be given every three hours. On the other hand, Rouff gives a drop of the first attenuation every evening; and Marcy gives from the first to the third attenuation. Ruddock gives a dose every ten or fifteen minutes during an attack; afterwards every three or four hours, and this is what I have been in the habit of doing for the past many years, using the lower triturations, say from the third to the sixth decimal, during the attack and the twelfth during the interval. I would add that I have found the triturations of the powdered root much more effective than dilutions of the mother tincture."

I also believe the triturations of the powdered root far superior to the dilutions of the tincture. In the so called "hay asthma." insufflation of the first and second decimal triturations of the root every two hours will be found of great value in subduing the attack.

> **IODIUM**—Scrofulous, cachectic people having a remarkable and unaccountable sense of weakness and loss of breath on going up stairs; skin dark brown; hypertrophy of the thyroid gland; women whose mammæ dwindle away; mammæ lose their fat and hang down heavily; extremely weak during menstruation, especially when going up stairs; long lasting uterine hæmorrhages; corrosive leucorrhea; chronic hoarseness; great emaciation, with night sweats and debility; symptoms aggravated by warm air and relieved by cold.

This is a grand constitutional remedy in chronic cases that are engrafted upon a low, cachectic scrofulous constitution, with much emaciation, night sweats and profound debility, especially when going up stairs; nutrition is extremely bad, and the lymphatic glandular system greatly enlarged.

Baehr says: "Iodium is one of those agents which, among it's symptoms of slow poisoning, numbers asthma as one of it's constant phenomena. In our *materia medica* these effects of Iodium are pointed out very imperfectly, and the reader is very much disposed to combine the symptoms pointing to asthma with the symptoms denoting inflammation. In the 'Deutsche Klinik' of 1856, three cases of Iodine asthma are recorded, which are of considerable interest. The asthma sets in after a protracted use of Iodine, whereas an acute intoxication with Iodine never causes asthma; the paroxysm sets in towards evenings, or, more commonly, about midnight, and lasts about half an hour; in one case it commenced with intense symptoms of laryngismus stridulus; the paroxysm was succeeded by excessive lassitude and an irresistible desire to sleep. Not withstanding the violent difficulties of breathing, every sign of a material change in the respiratory organs is wanting; there is emaciation without any increase of the secretions; great nervousness and restlessness during the intervals. Hence Iodine corresponds well with the purely nervous asthma, for which it has been prescribed more recently by several old school practitioners, of course in enormous doses. Except a few not very striking cases, homœopathic literature does not offer any cases of asthma successfully treated with Iodine."

A number of cases of laryngismus stridulus are reported in our journals that have been permanently cured with Iodium. It produces a tightness and constriction about the larynx, with much soreness and a hoarse, rasping voice. Frank relates a number of well marked, hard cases of chronic asthma cured with ten drop doses of pure Iodine.

"*Violent difficulty in breathing,* oppressed breathing, asthma with pain during deep inspiration, more violent and rapid beating of the heart, with a small, frequent pulse; *difficulty in expanding the chest when taking an inspiration; want of breath* when going up stairs; feeling of weakness in the chest and in the region of the heart; *sore pain* in the chest during respiration and contact; suffocating catarrh; *congestion of blood to the chest,* with an inclination to inflammation; *violent pulsations* in the chest, and palpitations of the heart, increased by every muscular exertion; *palpitations of the heart;* sensation as if the heart was being *squeezed together;* organic affections of the heart; burning and stinging tension in the muscles of the chest; hoarseness in the morning, with a deep, dry cough, and much tickling in the larynx."—*Hulls Jahr.*

It should be given by inhalation as wall as internally.

KALIUM HYDRIODICUM—Especially useful in scrofulous people who have been thoroughly saturated with mercury; in secondary and tertiary syphilis, and chronic rheumatism; mucous membranes of the mouth, lungs and kidneys chronically inflamed; fetid odor from the mouth, from ulceration of the mouth and fauces; ptyalism; chronic nasal catarrh in it's worst form; mucoid discharges from the urethra of both sexes; degeneration of the mucous membrances; mucous phthisis; purulent expectoration; exhausting night sweats and diarrhea; asthma in young people who are growing rapidly, have many rheumatic symptoms. The best remedy we have for chronic organic asthma; all forms of scrofula, swelling of the glands, chronic skin diseases, severe nocturnal bone pains; profuse, purulent secretions.

There is *no doubt* that this is the *best* remedy we have for chronic cases of organic asthma. No one remedy can compare with it, excepting Arsenicum; and doctors such as, Raue, Nichol, Baehr, Marcy and Hunt do not mention it when speaking of asthma.

Dr. W. B. Casey says of the *Iodide of Potassium:* "For a year past, I have looked through the various journals, in the expectation of seeing some thing on the subject of this article, but have not up to this time met with but a mere incidental mention of the fact that Hydro-iodide of Potash has been employed with some benefit in asthma. I therefore send you my experience with it, trusting that the statement which I make will excite the attention of our profession and lead to a trial of the remedy on a more extensive scale. Some two years since Prof. Mutter of Philadelphia, mentioned that he had accidentally discovered the fact to which I am now endeavouring to draw attention. I immediately commenced it's use with a number of patients suffering under this distressing and intractable complaint, and, to our mutual delight, they were all more or less speedily relieved. I have now made use of the medicine in some twenty five or thirty cases of asthma, some of them very severe and aggravated; and so far, where a fair trial has been made, it has not failed to afford unequivocal and decided relief. These facts I have stated at our county medical meetings, and have urged the adoption of the practice upon many of our neighbouring physicians; and so far as I can ascertain the result, all who have tried the remedy will indorse my statement of its value. I am happy to add the testimony of Dr. North, an eminent physician residing at Saratoga Springs who informs me that he has experienced in his own person great relief from the use of the medicine, and has witnessed the same effect in others. As a general rule, the patient is benefitted after a few days' employment of the drug, but some cases will require more time, perhaps weeks, before they improve; in one of mine, a very severe case, of over twenty years duration, I persevered for nearly three months before there was any decided amendment. I feared at the outset that the medicine would prove to be merely a palliative (and even then it would be invaluable), but further experience warrants my belief that,

ASTHMA

in mild cases of recent date, a cure may be effected. In almost one-fourth of my cases, relapses have occurred after discontinuing the remedy; this occurrence, however, was in most of them owing to severe attacks of catarrh, or to errors in diet, and consequent derangement of the digestive organs, which, by the way, should never be overlooked in the treatment of asthma. I may mention in this connection that most of my patients, while using this medicine, had an excellent appetite and gained flesh rapidly. A long continued use of the Iodide of Potassium will, in some subjects, occasion an eruption, generally of a pustular form (almost always ecthema); and I have twice been disposed to attribute to it the occurrence of a slight conjunctivitis; the omission of the medicine for a few days, together with a few doses of Rhubarb and Soda, will be found sufficient for the removal of these inconveniences. It would scarcely be worth while to offer, at the present time, my explanation of the *modus operandi* of this medicine in asthma. From two to five grains of Iodide of Potassium, given three times a day, dissolved in water or some syrup, as for instance that of Sarsaparilla or Tolu, will generally be found sufficient for ordinary cases of this disease. It's continuance must be regulated by the circumstances of each case; of course no intelligent practitioner need be reminded of the attention requisite as regards diet, clothing and exercise. It may not be uninteresting or irrelevant to mention that the Hydro-iodide has been given to several horses troubled with the heaves, and in all, while under the influence of the medicine, the disease was suspended. Hydro-iodide of Potassium is the basis of Whitcomb's notorious remedy for asthma."

Not withstanding this is old school testimony, I thought it too good to leave out. Dr. E.M. Hale says; "The best cures I ever made, remarkable both for promptness and permanency, were brought about by the following:

Kali hydriodicum ½³.

Fowler's Arsenical Solution, 13.

Aqua destillata, 13.

Give ten drops, three times a day in chronic cases, or every one, two or three hours in acute." I have tested this prescription, and can vouch for it's *great* utility.

Dr. Ruddock says: "*Kali hydriodicum*—This medicine is attended with marked success when prescribed in low attenuations, from ø to 3× and *persevered in.*"

SYMPTOMS : —Severe coryza; nose red and swollen, with profuse, watery nasal discharge; constant sneezing; dry, hard, hacking cough, afterwards accompanied by a copious, greenish expectoration; great oppression of breathing, with loss of voice; suffocative oppression and arrest of breathing; the constriction of the chest is so great that the lungs can not be inflated by the greatest effort of the patient; aggravated by rest; patient must move about to get relief; the dyspnea is so distressing, that the patient declares he will die. In chronic cases there is often a large secretion of mucus in the lungs which, when expectorated, has a green appearance, from having been secreted for a long time.

Auscultation reveals an immense amount of bronchial spasm, as indicated by the whistling, wheezing noises all over the chest.

There is a good deal of emaciation and debility, accompanied with many rheumatic symptoms about the body and in the chest.

Has sharp, violent stitches in the chest; sometimes the pains seem as if they would cut the chest in pieces.

ASTHMA

Adapted to both dry and humid asthma, but acts better in the dry form.

The first decimal triturations will, as a rule, be found all that is necessary, but when obstinate, I do not hesitate to dissolve twenty grains of the crude drug in twenty spoonsful of water, and give one spoonful as a dose, three times a day, in chronic cases; in acute, every two hours until relieved.

All the salts of Potash have a powerful influence over the lungs, and are of great utility in the treatment of asthma, especially the Kali nitricum and the Kali bichromium; also Kali bromatum and Kali carbonicum should be carefully studied.

> **LACHESIS MUTUS**—Sleeping greatly aggravates the symptoms; patient always distressed after sleeping; excessive sensitiveness of the throat, cannot bear the least touch of the finger; painful deglutition, regurgitation through the nose; women who are greatly troubled at climacteric with frequent flushings; cannot bear any pressure, not even the clothes, upon the uterine region, keeps constantly lifting them; great tendency to faint and insomnia; great sensitiveness of the larynx, when touched produces suffocation; dry, hard, spasmodic cough; sensation as it the lungs were being pressed up into the throat.

This remedy is adapted to the neurotic form of asthma, especially if it should occur in women at the climacteric age.

Dr. T. Nichol says: "Lachesis—the Belladonna of chronic diseases—is suitable to children suffering from hydrothorax, or where there is a largely bloated and lymphatic appearance; shortness of breath after a meal; tight breathing, dyspnea and oppression of breathing, with aggravation after eating; suffocative feeling in a recumbent position, or when touching the neck; spasmodic constriction of the chest, obliging the patient to rise from bed and to sit with the trunk bent forwards; slow and wheezing respiration; desire to take a deep breath, especially when sitting."

Pulte remarks that this remedy suits well after Arsenicum, and Laurie that it should be administered four hours after the third dose of Belladonna, when partial improvement only has resulted from the administration of the last named medicine.

> **LOBELIA INFLATA**—Spasmodic asthma, worse from exertion; feeling of weakness in the pit of the stomach; dyspnea with a feeling as if there was a lump in the œsophagus, rising into the mouth; excessive nausea and vomiting, with complete prostration after vomiting; sensation as if a thousand needles were pricking the skin; chronic vomiting in paroxysms.

Through the vagi this remedy has a powerful action upon the lungs, and is often of great value in arresting spasmodic asthma of recent origin. Cases especially calling for Lobelia are of the humid form and spasmodic in nature, with great irritation of the vagi.

Dr. T. Nichol says: "*Lobelia*—The practitioners of our school by no means agree as to the true sphere of this remedy in asthma, Dr. Marcy says that it 'is a remedy of great value in cases of spasmodic asthma induced by humidity, and certain other conditions of the atmosphere,' and Dr. Hughes states that 'in pure nervous asthma uncomplicated with bronchial irritation, Cuprum and Lobelia are most effectual.' Dr. Ruddock, who has had much experience in the disease, prescribes Lobelia in pure nervous asthma. Dr. Hempel thinks that it is undoubtedly homœopathic to some forms of spasmodic asthma; and Dr. Noack has arrived at the conclusion that it's operation is peculiarly directed to the pneumogastric nerve, an opinion which is strongly supported by both it's pathogenesis and it's curative effects. On the other hand, Hartmann, who is a great authority with the *middle aged* physicians of our

ASTHMA

school, says that 'this remedy seems to be principally adapted to asthma, depending upon degeneration of the bronchial mucous membrane, occasioned by chronic inflammation of the air passages,' while Baehr, a weighty authority, curtly remarks that 'Lobelia is more adapted to emphysema than to asthma.' Ruoff seems to be of the same opinion, for he directs Lobelia to be used in cases characterized by constant dyspnea increased by slight exertion, and aggravated by slight exposure to cold. My own experience is that the low dilutions meet the form of spasmodic asthma, to which the drug is homœopathic, while the medium and higher dilutions are adapted to a variety of the malady resulting from chronic inflammation of the air passages."

Hempel thus gives the key to the use of Lobelia: "Asthma, with irregular, jerking respiration, oppression, suffocative anxiety, as if the patient would die."

The attack is preceded or accompanied by a kind of prickly sensation through the whole system, even to the extremities of the fingers and toes; constrictive pain across the chest, and laborious breathing, with a disposition to keep the mouth open to breathe; oppression of the chest, causing a deep breath to be taken to relieve the pressive pain in the epigastrium, extending upwards to the chest, with or without cardialgia or pyrosis; much mucus in the throat; short, anxious and wheezing respiration, with spasmodic cough; nausea and vomiting, with great prostration, trembling of the limbs, with an intermittent pulse and cold sweat; burning sensation on passing urine, which is of a deep red colour and deposits a copious red sediment.

Many of our practitioners use the mother tincture exclusively, but Marcy recommends the potencies from the third to the sixth—a dose every two to four hours, as the symptoms require, and remarks that "I, myself, in common with many other practitioners, have seen very satisfactory results from Lobelia, not given as an emetic or depressant, but from the 2nd to the 6th dilution."

I have already given my views as to the dose.

> **LYCOPODIUM CLAVATUM**—Constant sensation of satiety, the least morsel of food causes a sensation of fulness up to the throat; great distention of the stomach and bowels with gas; much borborygmus, particularly in the left hypochondrium; long continued constipation, accompanied with much flatulence; copious sediment of red sand in the urine; humid asthma, there is much expectoration of mucus, or muco-purulent matter; night sweats and debility.

For long standing organic cases of humid asthma, where the digestion is greatly perverted, with excessive accumulations of flatus in the stomach and abdomen, no remedy is of more value. The Lycopodium asthma might well be called *flatulent asthma*, and the paroxysm is generally relieved by excessive eructations of flatus, or by a stool. In all probability the excessive asthmatic sufferings are reflex in the majority of cases; the great difficulty being caused by indigestion; but in tuberculosis Lycopodium is often *the* remedy.

> **MERCURIUS**—Scrofulous people, with induration of the glandular system; chronic nasal catarrh; profuse perspiration that does not relieve; teeth sore, loose, and the gums bleed easily; tongue coated white, thick and is heavy, with intense thirst; fetid breath; profuse flow of saliva; ulceration in the mouth and fauces; mucous, or muco-sanguinous stools, stools of blood; symptoms especially aggravated at night and in cold, damp weather; nightly bone pains; much jaundice; secondary syphilis.

In many cases of asthma, where there is a deep seated organic disease at it's foundation, Mercury will be found of great value, and especially if there is a long standing bronchitis present. With great discharge of mucus from the lungs, the Iodide of Mercury will be found an absolute specific in such cases.

Hartmann says: "Asthmatic paroxysms originating from the inhalation of the vapor of arsenic are removed by no other remedy with more certainty than by Mercurius 3d in repeated doses.

"Mercurius is also of great benefit in those" cases where smoking tobacco and cold air lessens the attack—Raue.

The *Cyranuret of Mercury* will often be the most useful form to use, especially where the bronchi are loaded with tough mucus.

> MOSCHUS—Nervous, hysterical asthma; Neurotic palpitations of the heart. Spasmodic hiccough; profuse urination; much thirst and great emaciation; patients inclined to be constantly cold and chilly.

This remedy is adapted to nervous, suffocative asthma, in hysterical subjects.

Dr. T. Nichol says; "Moschus is useful in the acute asthma of children, caused by exposure to cold, especially when the patient is of a nervous temperament. There is a violent feeling of constriction in the throat as if the glottis were involved in the attack, with a sense of spasmodic constriction in the windpipe and upper part of the bronchial tubes. This constriction increases until it becomes a suffocative spasm of the lungs which drives the patient to despair. Sometimes there is no cough present, but merely a little irritation at the commencement of the paroxysm, occasionally the cough is more marked. Noak and Trinks recommend Moschus to be given in doses of one grain of the first, second and third trituration, once or twice a day."

Frank has made some fine cures with Moschus.

> **NAJA TRIPUDIANS**—Has a powerful action upon the vagi, producing violent asthma and palpitations of the heart. Is of great value in asthma complicated with heart disease; *neurotic* symptoms predominate.

This remedy has a specific and powerful action upon the pneumogastric nerves, through it, violent suffocative asthma and palpitations of the heart are produced.

M. Preston M.D. of Norristown says, "I have used *Naja* in hay fever with every gratifying results, after the sneezing stage has passed and asthmatic troubles remain. I think it will not only prove of great value in relieving attacks of the subsequent asthma, but also prevent the annual recurrence of this great summer and autumnal pest."

"In asthma it has done one signal service and has exhibited power over some old and protracted, cases where all other medicines had failed to touch, and had been well nigh abandoned."

He uses the 30th potency.

SYMPTOMS:- Grasping at the throat with a sense of choking.

- Constriction and dryness of the throat.
- Choking, strangling and loss of breath after repose or sleep.
- Asthmatic constriction of the chest.
- Short hoarse cough, with a raw feeling in the larynx and upper part of the trachea.
- Dark red colour of the fauces and a livid face.
- Membranous croup, with difficult, rasping respiration and expectoration of membranous masses from the larynx.

NITRICUM ACIDUM—Asthma depending upon some virulent poison in the system, such as syphilitic, mercurial and scrofulous *miasm*; debilitated old people, with diarrhea; ulceration of the mucous membranes, especially of the mouth and throat; putrid breath ; tendency to diarrhea; fissures of the anus that produce great suffering during stool; intolerably offensive urine, smells like that of horses; bad effects of mercury; people with dark complexion, black hair and eyes, with a great tendency to take cold; ulcerations, that have a sensation as if a sharp splinter was being run into the ulcer at the slightest touch. Aggravations in the after part of the night.

This is an admirable remedy for asthma in patients that have had their systems filled with mercury, or have suffered from the effects of secondary syphilis, especially if they are scrofulous subjects.

Dr. Hartman says : "Nitricum acidum is an excellent remedy to eradicate the asthmatic disposition. It is particularly useful in delicate constitutions, persons with sensitive nerves and irritable temperaments, particularly when the organism has been weakened by mercurial treatment, or by syphilitic, scrofulous or hepatic diseases. The patient complains of fluent coryza, roughness of the throat, husky voice; as the coryza diminishes, the chest feels oppressed; if the coryza disappears entirely, the oppression increases to complete loss of breath, attended with palpitations of the heart and anxiety on ascending an eminence; or the patient complains of constant dyspnea; he is scarcely able to breathe, worse on leaning backward; sometimes the dyspnea is attended with anxiety, particularly when walking fast; when reaching the most violent degree, the disease increases to a spasmodic oppression of the chest, with rush of blood to the heart, languor, anguish, which is excited by the least emotion."

> **NUX VOMICA**—Choleric, sanguine, malicious, irritable people, who make great mental exertions; asthmatics who are used to an excess of stimulating drinks, highly seasoned food and have lived a sedentary life; frontal headache as if the eyes would be pressed out the head, with great irritability, everything offends; very dyspeptic, sour acid stomach constantly, much flatulency; constipation, with frequent, but ineffectual urging to stool; afflicted constantly with hæmorrhoids; dry coryza; dry spasmodic cough with much soreness in the epigastrium; symptoms greatly aggravated at 3 A.M.

Nux vomica asthma, might well be termed as a *dyspeptic asthma*, for the gastric symptoms always predominate, and the asthma is of a dry, spasmodic nature depending upon the reflex excitability of the vagi.

Dr. T. Nichol says : "Nux vomica is decidedly the leading remedy when the innervation of both branches of the pneumogastric nerve—it's gastric as well as it's pulmonary portion—is alike vitiated, and then the dyspepsia and the asthmatic affections are inseparable parts of one whole. Here as Dr. Satter remarks, the dyspeptic symptoms are the manifestations of the gastric portion of this deranged innervation and the asthma of the pulmonary portion of it, and in such cases Nux vomica is at once suggested to the mind of the practitioner. Dr. Ruddock remarks : "Nux is probably the best anti-spasmodic remedy. It is homœopathic to that condition of the digestive system which is the most common cause of irritation which results in bronchial spasm. Nux vomica is about the best curative medicine we have for simple spasmodic asthma, where there is no bronchial lesion, but a standing reflex excitability of the pneumo-gastric to impressions from without or through the stomach. One of the early cases which made Hahnemann famous, was of this kind, and Nux was given in material doses. Dr. Kidd also states that he considers it our best anti-asthmatic." While the gastric

ASTHMA

origin of Nux asthma is often unmistakably evident, the paroxysm itself often depends upon congestion of the lungs, and it is a characteristic symptom that *the oppression is more troublesome than the spasmodic symptoms.*

The attack is almost invariably preceded by symptoms of congestion in the lungs; nightly attacks of suffocative tightness especially in the lower part of the chest, accompanied by disagreeable or anxious dreams; shortness of breath on moving; constriction of the chest, with want of air on going to bed; hacking pain and anguish in the region under the heart and in the region of the hypochondria; tension and pressure in the chest, which seems to be constricted in it's transverse direction. The cough is short and hacking with difficult expectoration, which becomes looser towards morning, or the cough may be dry and concussive. It is a characteristic sign that the lower part of the thorax is almost immovable, while the abdominal respiration is quite marked. The abdomen, especially in the region of the stomach, is much distended with flatulence, accompanied by bitter or acid eructations and gripping or contractive pains. The dyspnea is increased by physical exertion of almost any kind, by eating and by lying down in the evening. The asthma is diminished by reclining on the back, or on changing from one posture to another, or by turning from one side to another. The disposition is passionate and irritable, with frequent bursts of ill temper.

"After the paroxysm subsides it leaves a condition of the digestive organs for which Nux vomica is the great remedy. The tongue is coated with a thick yellow fur; there is often a slight nausea, flatulence and constipation. Besides the breathing is seldom quite right; generally there remains a sort of a physical memory of the struggle. The patient feels that no liberties must be taken either of diet or exercise. Out of this secondary state of bondage nothing will liberate so effectually as Nux vomica."—Dr. Russell.

Drs. Marcy and Hunt recommend the 3rd to the 6th dilutions to be used; Caspari the 12th; but Dr. Bayes thinks that the dilutions from the 6th to the 30th act better than the lower, an opinion with which the present writer heartily agrees.

> **OPIUM**—Reflex asthma, the disease originates from some lesion of the brain; sopor and general symptoms of paralysis of the brain; extreme drowsiness and coma; face purplish and swollen; constipation; stools composed of round, hard, black balls; paralysis of the sphincter muscles; dry, spasmodic, titillating cough, greatly aggravated at night; scanty expectoration; bed feels so hard he cannot lie upon it; frequent hot flushes, followed by cold, clammy perspiration; bad effects from fright.

Opium is only useful as a palliative during the paroxysm, in the reflex nervous form, the organic lesion producing the asthma being located centrically in the brain.

Dr. T. Nichol says: "Opium is by no means a remedy of the first rank, yet cases occur in which it affords very prompt relief, especially when fright has been the casue."

Kreussler says that "Opium and Ignatia rank with Nux vomica, with this difference, that they are more suitable to the milder forms of asthma, and for children rather than adults."

Baehr places opium among the remedies from which most may be expected during the attack itself. "Opium, especially, sometimes renders substantial aid without it being necessary to employ large doses on this account. Morphia, 2nd trituration, two or three grains at a dose, exerts a sufficiently powerful effect, and if this dose is not sufficient, the remedy can only do harm. A copious secretion of mucus always counterindicates Opium."

The pathological state may be either congestion of the lungs, (which is hardly entitled to be called asthma), or it

ASTHMA

may be spasm of the bronchial tubes, which is more properly entitled to that appellation, for Opium is capable of producing either of these states on the healthy, and is consequently capable of curing them in the sick. The breathing is deep, stertorous and rattling, with loud mucous ronchii in the chest, and extreme anguish from dread of suffocation. There is tightness of breath, with oppression and spasmodic constriction of the chest suffocative fits during sleep like nightmares, with very difficult breathing during sleep. The cough is dry and suffocative, with a bluish redness of the face and dryness of the skin.

I would be positively afraid to give the enormous doses mentioned by Baehr—"Morphia, second trituration, two or three grains at a dose"—but have seen fine results from the twelfth trituration and the thirtieth dilution, given not as a mere palliative, but as a true curative remedy.

Morphine is often a valuable palliative, and the physician need not fear the effects of one-eighth, or in some cases even one quarter of a grain at a dose. These large doses will ward off the, so called, hay asthma entirely in some people. I know one physician who could not practice during fall without Morphine to ward off asthma.

> PHOSPHORUS—Tall, thin persons, with dark hair; long, slim, hard stool evacuated with a great deal of difficulty; diarrhea which pours out in great quantities like water from a hydrant, very exhausting, with a weak, empty, or gone feeling in the pit of the stomach; with this gone sensation in the stomach there is often great heat between the shoulders; hard, tight, dry cough, which racks the patient and is very exhausting; great sexual desire or impotence; obstinate hæmoptysis; slight wounds bleed much; degeneration of the brain and liquefaction of the spinal cord.

This is a valuable remedy in chronic organic cases of asthma in tall, slender people, that are greatly troubled with a weak, gone sensation in the epigastric region, with a strong phthisical habit.

Dr. T. Nichol says : "Phosphorus, to the mind of the homœopathic practitioner, calls up the idea of pneumonia rather than asthma, but it is really a valuable remedy against the latter malady. Ruoff and Pulteboth give the pathological indication 'phthisical habit'—and this is the leading idea of Phosphorus in asthma of children. The breathing is noisy and panting, and the dyspnea is marked; the oppressive breathing and oppression of the chest are aggravated in the evening and morning, also when sitting or during exercise; great oppressive anxiety in the chest; stridulous inspirations in the evening, when falling asleep; nightly suffocative paroxysm, as if paralysis of the lungs was threatened; spasmodic constriction of the chest; hoarse cough with saltish or sweetish expectoration, which is often blood streaked; stitches and sticking pains in the chest, with heaviness, fulness and tension. Constant chilliness is present, with languor and debility. In the cases in which Phosphorus has succeeded in my hands, the stethoscope revealed the presence of *congestion in the thorax* as a result of the spasm in the bronchial tubes and partial paralysis of the lungs. I have seen fine results from all preparations, from the 6th to the 200th, but feel surest of success when giving the 12th to the 24th dilution."

> **PULSATILLA PRATENSIS**—Very affectionate females, with blue eyes, blonde hair, inclined to be fleshy and easily excited to tears; symptoms are all aggravated in a close, warm room, and relieved in the open air; symptoms very changable, well one hour and miserable the next; bad taste in the mouth every morning, thickly coated tongue; stomach easily disordered from rich fat food; sour vomiting; gastrodynia; mucous diarrhea, catamenia too late and scanty; patient inclined to be chilly constantly; hard, racking, loose cough that makes the stomach sore, every coughing fit causes water to be emitted from the bladder; flying rheumatic pains, with much chilliness; chlorosis.

Humid asthma, especially in women with menstrual disturbances, is the great field for the use of Pulsatilla.

Hartmann says: "If an asthmatic spasm be caused by the vapor of sulphur, Pulsatilla is the best remedy to stop it; it is likewise the best remedy for asthma caused by the abuse of sulphur water. I have frequently been led to give Pulsatilla by the good natured, mild countenance of the patient, that seemed to invite pity, a reflex of the patient's character in his healthy days; it is likewise useful when the asthma depends upon hypertrophy of the pulmonary mucous membranes; this condition is recognized by the fact, that after the abatement of the paroxysm the patient is relieved by raising large quantities of disorganized mucus, after the discharge of which a physical examination reveals in many places the bronchial respiration, as in partial emphysema of the lungs; this kind of asthma might be termed asthma humidum. Pulsatilla is likewise useful in asthma senile and urinosum of old people, where the audible vesicular breathing points distinctly to œdema of the lungs and scattered interstitial tubercles. It is highly recommended in asthma menstruale and cardiacum of chlorotic and hysteric subjects."

The prominent gastric symptoms produce through sympathy great depression of spirits, melancholy, anxiety and great dread of suffocation. "Short suffocative and extremely difficult respiration, as if from want of sufficient air, or choked by some irritating substance; the patient is obliged to retain the erect posture; his movements are rapid, and his whole appearance indicates great distress and anxiety; tongue loaded with a thick coating; breath offensive; frequent eructations; hiccough; countenance pale, alternating with redness; attacks usually coming on at night, during sleep."

Use the low attenuations.

STANNUM METALLICUM—Profound prostration of strength; patient must drop down, but can get up very well; goes up stairs well, but becomes faint on coming down; talking or reading aloud produces great exhaustion; symptoms are, all relieved by menstruation; loose rattling cough, copious yellow or greenish expectoration, with a very weak feeling in the throat and chest.

This remedy is useful in chronic cases of humid asthma, with so much debility that the legs are not able to support the body, complicated with chronic bronchitis, with an abundant secretion of mucus, or genuine tuberculosis, second stage.

Baehr says: "Stannum may be tried if the attack supervenes during the existence of chronic catarrh, and the decrease of the attack is attended with a copious secretion of mucus."

Dr. T. Nichol says: "The precise phase of the malady for which Stannum has been thought suitable is when the attack supervenes during the existence of chronic catarrh, and the decrease of the attack is attended with a copious secretion of mucus. Oppression at the chest with mucous ronchus, and this oppression, which seems to be principally due to the large amount of mucus, is worse especially in the evening and at night, when lying down, also in the day time during every exercise, and frequently attended with anguish and a desire to remove the clothes. The cough is attended by copious expectoration of viscid, lumpy or saline taste. Noack and Trinks recommend one grain of the 2nd, 3rd or 6th trituration, once or twice daily."

SPONGIA TOSTA—Chronic hoarseness; dry, sibilant cough, with great dryness of the larynx; every secretion if perfectly tight and dry, without any mucous rattling sound, with suffocative breathing; must have the head high; goitre; indurated glands.

In organic cases of dry, spasmodic asthma, with severe dyspnea on lying down; exertion produces great exhaustion in the chest; sudden weakness while walking; much chilliness in the back; symptoms aggravated in a warm room, Spongia will be found of great value, in the 2nd and 3rd decimal trituration.

Baehr says : "Spongia has so far been found useful only in asthma depending on tuberculosis, but it has never effected a complete cessation, only a marked diminution in the frequency and intensity of the attacks. The paroxysm is characterized by a marked contraction of the glottis, a wheezing respiration, with complete loss of voice. In a few hours, the patient hawks up a substance resembling soaked sago."

SULPHUR—Constant heat on the top of the head; rush of blood to the head, with vertigo; has happy dreams, awakens singing; feels very weak and faint at 11 A.M., cannot wait for dinner; feeling of goneness in the pit of the stomach; chronic constipation from abdominal plethora, accompanied with bleeding hæmorrhoids; stools hard and knotty; excoriating morning diarrhea. In women, menses too early, too profuse and last too long; acrid, excoriating leucorrhea; catarrhal symptoms become worse and worse; feels suffocated, wants the windows and doors open; much rattling of mucus in the lungs; plastic pleurisy; frequent hot flushes, with faintness; much burning in the soles of feet, puts them out of bed to get them cool; vesicular eruptions upon the skin; chronic rheumatism.

Chronic cases of asthma, complicated with eruptive skin diseases; rheumatism or some constitutional taint; it may be either humid or dry, but generally the breathing and cough is neither loose nor dry, but half way between, of a wheezing character; there seems to be much mucus in the lungs, but none, or only a trifle, is expectorated; sensation, as if the lungs touched the back while coughing. Sulphur is adapted to nearly every kind of asthma, but is the most useful in the humid form.

Dr. T. Nichol sums up it's action as follows: "Sulphur is, according to Hartmann, 'a most universal remedy for asthma. There is scarcely a case where Sulphur is not used. It suits almost every constitution and temperament, and antidotes the bad effects of a number of metallic poisons.' Pulte says that it may be given in almost any acute or chronic attack of asthma, if several other remedies were insufficient; and Hughes remarks 'that in a great number of cases you will discover, on inquiry, gouty inheritance or proclivity, or, what is almost the same thing, some form of cutaneous disease alternating with the dyspnea. In these cases you will get most satisfactory results from Sulphur.' The paroxysms of asthma, almost suffocating, occur mostly at night, with fullness and weariness, burning or spasms in the chest; sometimes the asthma occurs during day time, even when walking in open air; contractive pain around the chest; periodical constrictive spasms in the chest, with a blue face and short breath, particularly in the evening, in a warm room; wheezing, mucous rattling; ronchus in the chest; oppressed breathing and suffocative fits, especially at night; suffocative cough, with spasmodic constriction of the chest and an urging to vomit; difficult expectoration of whitish mucus, or else copious yellow expectoration; spasms in the chest, with a compressive sensation and pain in the sternum; bluish-red face, short breath and an inability to speak. Kreussler remarks that 'Sulphur is suitable to scrofulous, rickety and psoric individuals, especially with a warm skin, internal heat and hurried pulse; whereas Calcarea has a cool, brittle skin, and a sluggish pulse.' As to the dose, Hughes says that 'you may send your patients to a sulphurous spring, and Dr. Russell recommends the same; but I think they will do nearly as well at home under the usual potencies of the drug, of which I prefer the lowest.'"

My experience is the opposite of this. Among the few cases of medicinal aggravations which I have seen, were several

ASTHMA

of asthma, aggravated by the use of Sulphur in doses of the 3rd and 4th decimal triturations, and I have noticed the finest results from the 12th trituration to the 30th dilution.

TARTAR EMETIC—Large collections of mucus in the bronchial tubes, expectorated with great difficulty, indicating approaching paralysis of the vagi; coughing produces a sound as if there was a mouthful of mucus about to run over in the lungs; paralysis of the lungs, with great dyspnea and fits of suffocation; œdema of the lungs; much nausea and vomiting of mucus; very thirsty; colliquative diarrhea; lumbago.

This is a very valuable remedy in acute cases of humid asthma complicated with catarrh of the lungs. My friend, Dr. T. Nichol, says : "Tartar emetic has been comparatively used little in asthma, yet both Jahr and Laurie remark that it is frequently of great service in the asthma of children, while Hartmann says that plethoric asthma is perhaps the more immediate sphere of action for this agent. The suffocative distress, with anxious oppression and shortness of breath, depends partly upon the constriction of air passages and partly upon a low grade of inflammation in the bronchial tubes, accompanied by an excessive secretion of mucus. The malady is aggravated in the evening or in the morning, in bed, and is relieved by sitting up. Choking and retching are also present, with nocturnal paroxysms of suffocation accompanied by loud wheezing and rattling in the chest. Congestion of blood to the lungs is a frequent pathological state with palpitations of the heart, and the anguish is sometimes increased by sudden, violent beats of the heart, as if it would start out of it's place. Hartmann remarks that though there are occasional palpitations between the paroxysms, yet no organic disease could be discovered, showing that Tartar emetic suits asthma, with or without organic affections of the heart.

As to the dose, Noack and Trinks advise one grain of the 1st, 2nd or 3rd trituration, to be given once or twice daily. In my own practice I have usually dissolved a grain of the 3rd or 4th decimal trituration, in 12 teaspoonfuls of water, and given a teaspoonful every half hour during the attack, and every two hours during the interval."

> **VERATRUM ALBUM**—Great drops of cold sweat upon the forehead, with anguish and fear of death; cerebral congestion, with a bloated bluish face; much vertigo; cold, collapsed, pinched up face, violent nausea, and vomiting, exhausting diarrhea with violent colic; intense thirst for cold water; cold tongue and breath; brought on by ice cream and cold drinks; great prostration.

The action of this remedy is quite similar to Tartar emetic, and is especially useful in cases of humid asthma of great violence, the oppression and suffocation being of such intensity that it would seem as though the patient would die.

Dr. Nichol says: "Veratrum album is a well known remedy for inveterate asthma, especially when the spasmodic symptoms predominate. The asthmatic symptoms are very violent, even when sitting erect and during exercise, with pains in the side and hollow cough. Great prostration is present, with a small, slow, intermittent pulse, coldness of the skin, especially of the nose, ears and feet; nausea and vomiting before and after the attack, which is accompanied by cold perspiration. Laurie makes the remark that Veratrum should be administered four hours after the third dose of China, when the last named medicine has been productive of inadequate benefit (a phantasy), and several authors point out that it suits well after Ipecac and Arsenicum."

ASTHMA

> **VERATRUM VIRIDE**—Intense cerebral congestion, feeling as though the head would burst open; with nausea, vomiting and singing in the ears; livid colour of the face; nose pinched, cold and blue; cold sweat on the forehead; sudden nausea and vomiting of glairy mucus; the least quantity of food produces violent vomiting; intense and violent spasmodic asthma; myalgia.

As a palliative in violent, acute cases of spasmodic asthma, accompanied by intense congestion of blood to the lungs; the oppression of the respiratory organs being so great that the patient cannot lie down for days, for fear of suffocation, with a wheezing, rattling, loose cough, but the sputa is raised with great difficulty. No remedy in the *materia medica* can equal *Veratrum viride,* and to get it's best effects, it must be given in nauseating doses, of Squibb's Fluid Extract, two drops at a dose every half hour, until three to six doses are given, and then one drop at a dose, every one or two hours to the point of relief, when an organic remedy should be substituted that is homœopathic to the case. If the patient is a child, the medicine should be given just half as strong.

I have just cured a case of spasmodic asthma, in a gentleman who has been subject to the disease every fall and winter for years, the attacks lasting for weeks at a time. At this particular period he had not lain down for the space of two weeks; the breathing was very laborious and only accomplished in the sitting posture, accompanied with a hard racking, loose sounding cough, but the sputa was raised with great difficulty and with great wheezing in the lungs. In three days he was entirely relieved of the asthma, when he was ordered cod liver oil, and discharged convalescent.

There are a great number of remedies besides those mentioned that may be found useful in asthma, such as Arnica, Antimonium crudum, Cod liver oil, Colchicum, Cyclamen, Eupatorium perfoliatum, Glonoinum, Hydrocyanicum acidum,

Hyoscyamus, Kalium bichromicum, Sepia, Sabadilla, Sanguinaria, Silphium lacinatum, Thuja, Zincum, etc., etc.

We believe enough has been pointed out to meet all ordinary cases; if not, the reader is referred to our great *materia medica* for further assistance.

PRACTICAL EXPEDIENTS

Coffee—This is often of great value as a palliative; to be effective it should be taken as hot as it can be borne, as strong as it can be made, *"café noir,"* without milk or sugar, and on an empty stomach.

"Among stimulants, coffee, is perhaps the best known and the most generally efficacious. I find, in a majority of asthma cases I have treated, coffee has been tried, and it has given relief.

"Coffee taken with food not only does no good, but does positive harm by impeding the process of digestion. I have known more than one case, as I have mentioned elsewhere, in which coffee made in the ordinary way, and taken immediately after dinner, has a strong tendency to induce asthma, although, taken in the way I have above described, it had a very powerful beneficial influence.—*Dr. Reynolds' System of Medicine.*

STRAMONIUM—This is a remedy of great value as a palliative, either taken internally or by smoking, generally the latter method has proved the most successful. Smoking should be practised upon the first warning of a paroxysm, when relieved, morning and night, will often be enough for a few days.

ASTHMA

NITRATE OF POTASH—The smoke of burning nitre is one of the most useful palliatives we have. "A piece of blotting paper about the size of the hand, previously saturated in a solution of nitrate of potash, may be placed on a plate and ignited, when the fumes diffuse throughout the room, their influence soon becomes evident. A warm saturated solution of saltpetre, into which the patient can dip the paper himself, answers the purpose equally well. Many patients go to sleep habitually amid these nitrous fumes with a certainty of a sound, undisturbed rest; others have the papers in readiness wherever they go, and usually obtain relief from a few minutes inhalation of the fumes.

Inhaling the fumes of amyl nitrate is another means which sometimes gives speedy relief. But in adopting any of these expedients, ventilation must not be neglected; the windows should be regularly thrown wide open to renew the air of the apartment."—*Dr. Ruddock.*

TOBACCO—In a few cases, smoking tobacco, if the patient is not accustomed to it's use, will be found of service. The smoking should be continued until it produces slight nausea and faintness, but not continued long enough to produce vomiting.

CHLORAL HYDRATE—Will often act like a charm. Given in doses, large enough to produce sleep, generally fifteen or twenty grains, and repeated once in four hours, this remedy will be found quite efficacious, but it's action must be watched by a careful physician.

CHLOROFORM OR ETHER—These remedies will relax the contracted muscular fibres with great rapidity, and give immediate relief. No one but a physician should administer them, as, if entrusted to the patient, their use will be too frequently indulged in, and the patient's life may be sacrificed.

In the use of chloroform it is not required to produce a high degree of anesthesia. A few drops from the palm on the hand may suffice, which may be repeated several times until the dyspnea is subdued.

CARBONIC ACID GAS—Sir J. B. Simpson says : "I have often seen patients suffering from different forms of asthma, greatly relieved, and sometimes completely cured of their attack by being made to breathe carbonic acid gas, developed in an ordinary beer bottle, from a mixture of equal parts by measure of crystalized bicarbonate of soda and tartaric acid, with about a tumbler full of water, and inhaled through an India rubber tube, or through a narrow opening in the cork. The anesthetic cough is very striking."

DRY CUPPING—Two or three cups placed over the chest, has been found of signal sevice.

RUM—Many inveterate cases of asthma have yielded in one week's time by the use of rum. It is generally taken when going to bed at night, one or two tablespoonsful in a little syrup, or it may be used in water. Frank reports nine radical cures with rum. In these cases the lungs and mucous membranes of the digestive tracts were loaded with slimy mucus.

OZONIZED WATER—A wine glassful every three hours, has been found to be a valuable palliative.

INSUFFLATION of several remedies has been tried and found of much value in the so called, "hay asthma." The second decimal trituration of Mercurius corrosivus, and the first trituration of the Sulphate of Quinine have been the most frequently used, I have used the first triturations of Ipecac and Sanguinaria with good effect. Many other remedies might be used in the same way.

ELECTRICITY *and animal magnetism,* have been recommended by some, but have not proven of much value.

Baehr speaks highly of compressed air, and Dr. Wood, in his "Practice," says : "Insufflation of the lungs by a pair of bellows is among the means which have been used with advantage.

Sinapisms of mustard mixed with the white of an egg will often give much relief. Prepared with the egg it will never blister the patient.

M. Rayer applies a solution of ammonia, by means of a roll of lint moistened with it, to the velum pendulum palati, for a few seconds, and with almost uniform advantage. The patient is at first seized with a feeling of suffocation which is followed by coughing and copious expectoration, and soon after with great relief.

A pailful of cold water dashed upon the shoulders of the patient has acted as a palliative. Hot foot baths have also been useful in arresting the paroxysm.

The smoking of *Sarsaparilla,* by means of a pipe has been highly extolled, and I would suggest that *Veratrum viride* be also tried by means of a pipe. The latter, as a general rule, is the best internal remedy we have as a palliative. I have every reason to suppose that by smoking the stem, leaves and root, especially the latter, it will prove a rival to Stramonium as a palliative in asthma. Immediate relief would undoubtedly follow the use of this plant by smoking.

In hay asthma, a teaspoonful of sea salt in a tumbler of water, sniffed up the nostrils, three times a day, has been of much service.

Counter irritation, by the *Lebenswecker,* over the chest, is a valuable adjunct, and especially in chronic cases, will be of great value in connection with internal medication.

HECTIC FEVER AND NIGHT SWEATS

These two symptoms are so blended together (night sweat being simply a continuation of hectic fever), and both arising in phthisis, from one and the same cause, suppuration, that their treatment is united.

The remedies most useful in hectic fever and night sweats will be found more fully treated upon under cough, hæmoptysis, asthma, emaciation and debility; but we will note down the leading remedies with some of the indications for the most useful.

1. The most useful and first to be thought of are : Arsenicum, Calcarea carbonica, China, Carbo animalis and vegetabilis, Hepar sulphuris, Lycopodium, Mercury, Silicea, Sulphur, Sulphuric acid, Phosphoric acid and Nitric acid.

2. Aconite, Bryonia, Belladonna, Cod liver oil, Ferrum, Iodium, Graphites, Crotalus horridus, Morphine, Sambucus, Sepia, Staphysagria, Rhus tox., Polyporus officinalis, Muriaticum acidum, Psorinum and the Oxide of Zinc.

ARSENICUM ALBUM—Great prostration; symptoms aggravated at night, especially after midnight; great emaciation; wants to be in a warm room; cannot lie down for fear of suffocation; highest degree of dyspnea; great anguish and restlessness; pains worse during rest, and burn like fire; great thirst for cold drinks; drinks little but often; constantly licking the dry, cracked lips;

HECTIC FEVER AND NIGHT SWEATS

tongue dry, brown or black; gangrenous aphthe; hot burning like fire; obstinate nausea and vomiting; watery diarrhea, with a cadaverous smell, scenting the whole room; acrid, corroding diarrhea or leucorrhea; general anasarca, waxy pale skin, with great debility; aggravations from cold air, relieved by warmth.

In the last stages of phthisis, with profuse debilitating night sweats, or alternating with a dry, hot skin, or with profuse sweating, Arsenicum will prove of great value. It will also be of much service in the night sweats of debility, especially if there is malaria at the foundation of the disease. In phthisis, the sputa is excessively fetid, cough inclined to be hard and dry. Cold air is very disagreeable to the patient. Anasarca and dyspnea are prominent symptoms.

CALCAREA CARBONICA—Scrofulous leuco-phlegmatic people prone to diseases of the mucous membranes. Imperfect assimilation of food to tissue. Dry, flabby skin, great emaciation, with a constant tendency to take cold. Children with large open fontanelles, with much perspiration standing in large drops on the head, wetting the pillow thoroughly during sleep; great fatigue on going up stairs, is out of breath and has to sit down. Feet constantly feel as if he had on cold, damp stockings. Women who menstruate too often, too profusely and lasting too long; cannot bear cold, damp winds, takes cold constantly. Profuse night sweats when suppuration is abundant.

This is one of the most valuable remedies we have in profuse night sweats from suppuration, especially if the perspiration predominates upon the upper portion of the body, and is brought on from the slightest exertion. The skin is extremely sensitive to cold air, the slightest draught produces chilliness with goose skin. Hectic fever with glowing heat and redness of the face; much thirst, with burning in the palms and soles. Tightness of the chest, with a frequent necessity to take a full breath. Profuse sweat early in the morning, one after the other, is very weary and anxious before the sweat breaks out.

The great characteristic of the Calcarea sweat, is that it is always more abundant early in the morning and is very exhausting.

> **CHINA**—The system has been debilitated by the loss of vital fluids, such as blood, semen, diarrhea, leucorrhea, or over lactation; symptoms are intermittent, worse every other day. Touching the affected parts, or motion produces intense neuralgia; long lasting congestive headache, aggravated by a draft of air, in the open air, and relieved by pressure. Yellow coated tongue with loss of appetite and longing for acids, or canine hunger; abdomen feels as if full of gas, and eructations give no relief; acid stomach, nocturnal diarrhea of water, or undigested food; jaundice, anasarca, intermittent neuralgia, aggravated by touch, cold air or motion.

This is a remedy of great value, probably one of the most useful we have for night sweats and hectic fever. The patient is greatly debilitated, either from malaria, or suppuration and he wakes up every morning with his linen soaked with perspiration, but it affords no relief. With the debilitating sweats there is much thirst. And from the great loss of fluids, there is great sensitiveness of the skin, has a chill, followed by long continued heat and profuse perspiration.

> **CARBO ANIMALIS**—Scrofulous people with enlarged glands, indurated glands of a scirrhous nature, with fetid discharges, accompanied with extreme debility. Earthy coloured face, with copper coloured spots on the face and body; bleeding gums, with a sore, empty feeling at the epigastrium extreme debility attends the menstrual nisus and female diseases; acrid leucorrhea; offensive, acrid lochia; hypertrophy of glands, cough with expectoration of greenish pus; the least exercise tires out the patient. Profuse perspiration in organic diseases, especially of the lungs.

HECTIC FEVER AND NIGHT SWEATS

My partner Dr. A. E. Small pointed out to me the great utility of this remedy in night sweats. Over the past three years, I have verified his statement several times. All the carbons such as Carbo vegetabilis, Lithanthrax, etc., are useful in night sweats, but none can equal Carbo animalis. The cases in which it is the most useful are those where profuse suppuration is going on, and the patient is drenched with perspiration whenever he falls asleep, and the sweats are accompanied with extreme and profound prostration of the vital forces (See *Cough*.).

LYCOPODIUM CLAVATUM—Copious sediment of lithic acid gravel, resembling brick dust in the urine, excessive and constant accumulation of flatulence in the stomach and bowels; constant sensation of satiety, the least morsel of food causes a sensation of fulness up to the throat; much borborygmus, especially in the left hypochondrium; excessive constipation; slow depraved digestion; hectic fever; cough day and night, raising large quantities of mucus and pus; symptoms aggravated at 4 P.M.; gray yellow colour of the face.

In organic diseases of the lungs with night sweats that are copious, cold, clammy and sour, smelling like onions, with emaciation of the upper part of the body, while the lower portion is enormously distended; is extremely flatulent; nearly all his troubles are in sympathy, with depraved digestion, as shown by the constant and excessive accumulation of flatulence in the stomach and abdomen.

My friend and colleague Dr. D. A. Gorton of Brooklyn, N. Y., says: " This drug deserves honorable mention in connection with remedies for morbid sweats, my experience with the remedy allies it with Mercurius, and I seek it's aid under conditions of similar character. Lippe says the perspiration of Lycopodium "is frequently" cold, smelling sour, offensive, like onions or of blood. Jahr attributes to the drug, "Nocturnal sweats, often fetid or viscid, principally on the chest and back, cold sweat on the feet, sometimes copious and with excoriation of the skin." It has been most serviceable to me in the treatment of fetid perspiration in the axillæ and of the feet, accompanied with burning in the soles, in women suffering from chronic endometritis and disordered vaginal discharges. Potencies, the 30th and the 200th.

> **HEPAR SULPHURIS**—In all diseases where suppuration is inevitable; the slightest injury causes suppuration; the system has been poisoned with mercury; cannot bear to be uncovered, coughs as soon as any part of the body is uncovered; much hoarseness, has a loose, rattling, choking cough, with copious expectoration of mucus and pus; chronic hepatization of the lungs, with a constant tendency to perspire, especially upon the chest and head; in phthisis, sweats day and night without relief; the skin is excessively sensitive to take cold at very change in the atmosphere.

In phthisis or any other disease with profuse suppuration, Hepar sulphuris is one of the remedies most frequently called for. The patient sweats day and night without relief, and the perspiration is extremely acid, as noted by the sour smell that is constantly emitted. When there is ulceration of the lungs, it is accompanied with much rattling of mucus, suffocative attacks of breathing; the expectoration is more copious in the morning than in the evening; the patient cannot bear the slightest draft of air, which produces a cold.

> **SILICEA TERRA**—Chronic suppuration, especially in children with large bellies, weak ankles and much perspiration about the head; patient constantly wants to uncover himself; has a wonderful control over the suppurative process, seeming to mature abscesses when desired; great lack of vital heat, is cold and chilly all the time; obstinate constipation—the rectum has no power to expel the fecal matter, and the stool recedes after having been partially expelled; caries of the bones, and chronic suppuration in the joints; extremely fetid foot sweat; assails the nutrition rather than the functions of an organ.

HECTIC FEVER AND NIGHT SWEATS

This is a remedy of great value in profuse, debilitating, fetid night sweats, dependent upon an organic disease that has passed into the suppurative process. The patient is constantly troubled with fetid foot sweat, and the feet are icy cold all the time; in phthisis, the hectic fever is followed by constant perspiration, very copious at night, attended with much prostration, a loose, rattling cough, great emaciation, loss of appetite, a constant tendency to take cold, nightly diarrhea, etc. Dr. Holcomb has used the 6,000 dilution with wonderful curative powers in the last stages of phthisis.

SULPHURICUM ACIDUM—Great debility, with sensation of tremors all over the body, without trembling; aphthae, attended with much pain, coldness and relaxed feeling in the stomach, with loss of appetite and great debility; diarrhea with excessive debility; hæmorrhages from all the outlets of the body, of a dark blood; constant hot flushes at climacteric; feels that everything must be done in a great hurry; general debility.

This is the standard remedy for profuse night sweats in allopathic practice. It is more especially called for in profuse morning sweat, affecting principally the, upper part of the body, and accompanied with excessive and extreme debility. The old school gives from twelve to twenty minims at a dose, three or four times a day, of the dilute Sulphuric acid. The second and third decimal dilutions in our hands will yield fine results.

PHOSPHORICUM ACIDUM—People who have been weakened by the loss of animal fluids; by excesses, acute diseases, or a long succession of moral emotions; painless, watery diarrhea, with rumbling in the abdomen, and excessive accumulation of flatus; undigested stools; bad effects from sexual abuse; spermatorrhea; impotence; great apathy, and indifferent to all about him, can hardly be persuaded to speak; cerebral weakness from brain fag.

This is a remedy of great value in night sweats from general debility, from the loss of vital fluids, attended with great apathy and general prostration; not so valuable in night sweats from suppuration. The perspiration is cold and clammy.

> **NITRICUM ACIDUM**—Diseases depending upon some virulent poison, such as syphilitic, mercurial and scrofulous miasms, secondary syphilis, with mucous patches, and tubercles; easily bleeding ulcers, herpes, condylomata, salivation from abuse of mercury, spreading ulcers in the mouth and throat; mouth full of fetid ulcers; sore throat, discharging a thin purulent matter; diarrhea, with great pain in the anus, as if it was fissured; painful diarrhea, with profuse discharge of blood; proctalgia; urine smells like horses' urine and is extremely offensive; in women, violent pressure as if the womb was going to be forced into the world; bloody leucorrhea; lean people, with a bilious temperament, who take cold easily; a prominent key for it's use is a feeling, as if a sharp splinter was being stuck into the affected part; symptoms are aggravated at night, especially after midnight.

For old, broken down constitutions, with syphilis, or for those suffering from the effects of mercury, attended with much debility and profuse perspiration at night, smelling extremely fetid, like horses' urine, Nitricum acidum will be found the best remedy we have for such a state, and we will be only too glad to give it a fair showing. To get it's full benefit it must be given in the first or second decimal dilutions, prepared in water.

Dr. Gorton says: "Nitricum acidum is an invaluable remedy in those dyscrasic conditions in which the blood is impoverished and the secretions foul, with weakness of the vital powers. I have used it for foul smelling perspiration of the feet with gratifying results, also for sweating hands with a sourish smell accompanied with a fetid and excoriating leucorrhea, as well as sweat on the feet, sometimes fetid, with excoriation between the toes. To get it's best effects it must be given in appreciable doses.

> MERCURIUS SOLUBILIS—Symptoms are greatly aggravated at night, and in cold, damp weather; profuse perspiration gives no relief; much enlargement of the glandular system; teeth very soft, loose, and feel too long; much bleeding from the gums; salivation, with excessive fetor of breath; red tongue; the mucous membrane of the whole buccal cavity and tongue is covered with aphthous ulcers, salivary glands greatly enlarged, accompanied with profuse flow of saliva; intense thirst; mucous, serous or bloody diarrhea; jaundice; nocturnal bone pains.

In the last stages of tuberculosis, with ulceration of the lungs, accompanied with aphthous ulceration of the mucous membrane of the mouth and intestinal tract, this remedy is the most useful and reliable one that the physician can command. The perspiration is general, cold and clammy, leaving a yellow stain on the linen, continues most of the time, but much worse at night, especially during sleep; accompanied with heat and chilliness alternately. The sweat is apt to be very offensive. The Mercurius solubilis and vivus act best upon women and children, while the corrosivus acts best upon men.

PRACTICAL EXPEDIENTS

BATHING, the use of water in arresting night sweats cannot be omitted by the physician, for the benefical results which follow bathing and friction of the skin are so prompt and marked that the patient after commencing it's use could not be induced to omit his bath; as a rule a warm bath is to be preferred, the temperature of which should be 90° to 95° F.; if above this, 98° to 112° it will have the opposite effect, producing profuse perspiration and great prostration, but if taken from three to six degrees below the normal temperature of the body, once or twice a day, followed by vigorous friction with a crash towel or flesh glove to get a complete reaction, it will not only arrest the tendency to night sweats, but forms the best protection we have against the liability to frequent colds. It's duration should be from fifteen to thirty minutes according to the strength of the patient.

Many patients cannot bear the shock of fresh water; in such cases, a handful of common salt or *sea salt*, thrown into the bath will obviate the chill, and the patient will be greatly benefited by the bath; the saline matter which the water holds in solution acts as a stimulant to the skin, enlivening the feeble circulation. relieving the cold hands and feet and the general chilly condition of the body. In strong, vigorous patients, the cool bath, lasting from three to five minutes, with water at a temperature of 60° to 75°, will tone up the body with great rapidity; but if continued too long, instead of tonic effects, great depression will follow, and much injury will be done; when the patient is too weak to take a full bath, sponging the body three or four times a day with salt and water, soap and water, vinegar and water or alcohol, followed by vigorous friction, will not only be a great comfort to the patient, but of much value in arresting the night sweats and toning up the functions of the skin glands. The external use, in water, of the remedy homœopathic to the case will often be of great value in aiding the action of it's medicinal effects. Bathing the body immediately after eating should never be practised, but the bath should be taken one hour before eating or four hours after, so as not to interfere with the process of digestion, by drawing the blood from the digestive organs to the skin.

A warm glow and exhilaration of spirits after the bath indicates it's beneficial action and on the contrary, chilliness and depression are indications of harm, and a bath should not be taken.

Dr. C. J. B. Williams in his work on consumption, treating of night sweats says : "When the perspiration is only slight, sponging the chest with toilet vinegar or dilute sulphuric acid at night is sufficient; when more profuse a night draught of half a drachm of dilute nitro-hydrochloric, or sulphuric acid in glycerine and water, will often answer the purpose. Gallic acid in ten grain doses, once or twice a day, is an excellent remedy, and sometimes the addition of the tincture of perchloride of iron or the sulphate of quinine, to the daily tonic, will have the desired effect, but these two last drugs are apt to increase the cough, and must therefore be given with caution.

The medicine we have found to act almost as a specific on night sweats, is the Oxide of Zinc, in doses of two or three grains in the form of a pill at night. This we have given ourselves, and seen other physicians give to thousands of patients, and the good results have generally been so prompt and lasting, that only in a few cases has it been necessary to continue it's use for any length of time."

Hot alcohol or brandy is often of great service and comfort to the patient, used in the form of a sponge bath, followed by friction with a crash towel, coarse flannel or the flesh brush. If the perspiration is very profuse and debilitating the addition of Cayenne pepper, salt or mustard, will so stimulate the skin, that the night sweats will be soon controlled.

Lime water, if used externally, especially if *Calc.* is homœopathic to the case, will be found of great value.

Skimmed milk, a tumblerful taken at bed time, has often arrested night sweats, probably due to the lactic acid contained in the milk.

Koumiss, in all probability, will be found the most useful practical expedient the physician can resort to, it being the most nutritious and simple food the patient can take, it is absorbed into the blood almost as soon as taken; we believe that it alone, will cure the majority of cases we are called upon to treat; it should be used as a diet, from one to four pints daily (See *Koumiss*).

APHTHAE

In some cases of consumption this symptom gives the patient much suffering and requires the special attention of the physician. For it's treatment the following remedies deserve notice.

1. Mercurius, Chlorate of Potash, Borax, Argentum nitricum, Nitricum acidum, Sulphuricum acidum, Muriaticum acidum and Arsenicum.
2. Nux vomica, Sulphur, Aurum muriaticum, Carbolicum acidum, Gallicum acidum, Phosphoricum acidum, Calcarea carbonicum, Hydrastis, Natrium muriaticum, Iodium, Kalium hydriodicum, Lycopodium, Alum, Baptisia, Hepar sulphuris, Carbo vegetabilis, Staphysagria, Ammonium carbonicum, Cantharis and Kreosotum.

MERCURIUS SOLUBIUS—Affects especially the mucous membrane of the mouth; gums bleed and are inclined to ulcerate around the teeth, very fetid breath; red tongue with much burning and great thirst, mouth filled with aphthous ulcers. Profuse ptyalism, salivary glands greatly swollen; stools of mucus and blood; much perspiration that does not relieve. Aggravated at night and in cold, damp weather.

This is one of the most reliable remedies we have for aphthous ulceration of the mouth, not only when found in consumptives but in all cases where it's characteristic symptoms are prominent, such as in spongy, easily bleeding gums; swollen and painful, burning ulcers on the inside of the cheeks and tongue. Ptyalism, very fetid breath; general emaciation and prostration of strength, especially in the last stages of consumption, internally and locally. The first trituration of Merc. used locally will give great satisfaction.

> **KALIUM CHLORICUM**—Has a special action upon the buccal follicles of the mouth. Follicular ulcers upon the inside of cheeks and tongue. Aphthous ulcers cover the mouth; mouth filled constantly with saliva; glands enlarged and sore; gums inflamed and bleed; burning, stinging blisters on the tongue and buccal cavity; great heat in the mouth.

This remedy is as nearly a specific for stomatitis or aphthous sore mouth as can be found in the *materia medica*. If used locally and internally, but few cases will resist it's action. My favourite way of administering it is to let the patient put a small crystal in the mouth and suck it until all dissolved. By using a small crystal this way, every hour or two, the majority of cases will, in from one to three days, be effectually cured.

> **BORAX VENETA**—Aphthæ appearing suddenly; the whole buccal cavity covered with white fungous growths, limited to the mouth and fauces; great heat and dryness of the mouth; profuse mucous diarrhea; cannot bear downward motion; symptoms all aggravated in damp weather.

This is a remedy of much value, when in the first stage of phthisis, aphthæ suddenly make their appearance, completely filling the mouth in twenty four hours. The remedy may not only be given internally in the first three triturations, (I prefer the first two decimal triturations), but also used topically for a child, four grains to an ounce of water, and for an adult, ten grains to an ounce, applied locally every two hours will be found a serviceable application. Locally the first decimal trituration is of great value.

A good way to use Borax is to mix it with glycerine, using from thirty to forty grains of Borax to one ounce of glycerine; apply with a soft brush.

> **ARGENTUM NITRICUM**—Patient seems all withered and dried up; patient can't think, can't walk, can't talk, he gets so giddy; time seems hours to him, when it has only been a few minutes; is in a great hurry to do things; much flatulence, the stomach seems as if it would burst; fluids seem to run straight through the intestinal canal without stopping; green fetid diarrhea; much emaciation and debility, particularly in the lower extremities, with much chilliness.

In the last stages of tuberculosis this will be found of great value in the malignant form that has resisted all other remedies; the remedy is not only to be given internally, but every second or third day the solid stick should be used thoroughly over the entire diseased surface, especially if there is any deep ulceration. The caustic effect, in deep aphthous ulceration of the mouth, seems to have the power to set up at once healthy action in the diseased surface, and the ulcers heal rapidly.

> **NITRICUM ACIDUM**—If the disease is engrafted upon a person afflicted with mercurial or syphilitic poison; broken down constitutions from mercurial or scrofulous miasms; old people with much debility and diarrhea; salivation and ulceration of the mouth from abuse of mercury; spreading ulcers in the mouth and throat; putrid smelling breath; mouth filled full of fetid ulcers; bloody saliva; chronic inflammation of the fauces, extending up into the nose, with discharge of a thin, purulent matter; fissures of the anus, with chronic diarrhea; intolerable fetor of urine; suitable to lean people, broken down with mercury, and very liable to take cold.

The great field for the use of Nitricum acidum is in people who have been mercurialized; in such cases no remedy can equal it. The aphthous ulceration spreads rapidly, and is of the most fetid and disgusting nature; the slightest touch causes the ulcers to bleed profusely; gums spongy and bleed easily; teeth loose; the slightest touch causes a sensation in the ulcers as if sharp sticks were being thrust into them; great dryness and heat in the mouth and throat; tongue looks red, like a piece of raw beef.

I use the first and second decimal dilutions, prepared in water, five drops every two or four hours, and a gargle of the same every three hours.

> **SULPHURICUM ACIDUM**—Great exhaustion from some deep seated dyscrasia; great debility, with sensation of tremors all over the body, without trembling; profuse perspiration, with great debility; cold relaxed feeling in the stomach with great debility, constipation, with pricking pains in the anus during stool; hæmorrhages of black blood from all the outlets of the body; constant flushes at climacteric, with a tremulous sensation all over the body; menses too early and too profuse, always preceded by a distressing nightmare; patient feels as if everything must be done in a great hurry.

Mouth filled with aphthous ulcers, which are exceedingly painful to the patient, attended with a greatly increased secretion of saliva. In the last stages of tuberculosis, where the mouth is covered with aphthæ, sulphuricum acidum, applied twice a day, a few minutes at a time, with a spray producer, will be found of great value and a comfort to the patient; or it can be mixed with glycerine and applied with a camels' hair pencil; dilute sulphuric acid and water used as a gargle will also be of much value; internally I use the second and third decimal attenuations prepared in water.

MURIATICUM ACIDUM—Acts especially upon the mouth and anus; excessive dryness of the mouth and tongue, tongue is heavy and paralyzed; excessively foul breath, from sloughing ulcers in the mouth and throat; salivary glands inflamed, tender and swollen; diarrhea, the anus is so tender it cannot be touched; watery involuntary stools; putrescence of the body fluids; low fevers. In women, menses too early, too profuse, accompanied with great sadness; great sensitiveness to damp weather.

This acid is of great value in aphthous ulceration of the mouth in the last stages of consumption accompanied with great debility. The aphthous ulcers of the mouth and throat slough and tend to run together. Aphthæ in the last stages of tuberculosis denote great debility, and are often the harbinger of dissolution; consequently what we do has to be done at once. These mineral acids seem to tone up the body so rapidly that often a cure may be made when it would almost seem impossible. They should always be used locally as well as internally, especially if the disease is parasitical.

ARSENICUM ALBUM—Great prostration, with rapid sinking of vital forces; burning pain, the parts burn like fire; great anguish, restlessness and fear of death; intense thirst for cold water, drinks often but little at a time; cannot lie down for fear of suffocation; wants to be in a warm room; pains worse during rest, relieved by motion, great loss of flesh; anasarca and general dropsy; cadaverous diarrhea, with great tympanitis, abdomen burns like fire.

This remedy is adapted to the most malignant forms of aphthæ, might be called gangrenous, extending through the whole intestinal tract, attended with much burning distress, thirst, vomiting and exhausting diarrhea.

Marcy and Hunt say: "Stomatitis occurring in patients in malarious districts, most of whom have been injured by quinine; or where the water is more or less stagnant, and impregnated with the common causes of malarious fever. There is a depraved condition of the system analogous to typhus, the local eruption is vesicular in character; the edges of the tongue ulcerated, aphthæ, violent burning pains; swollen and readily bleeding gums, looseness of teeth; debility; sinking.

PRACTICAL EXPEDIENTS

A nutritious, but easily digested diet, to promote the general health of the patient, is the first thing to be done. Vegetable acids as found in oranges, lemons, apples, are often of great utility.

Where digestion is greatly at fault, Koumiss, one quart a day, will be found just what is wanted to restore the patient to health and strength again.

Dr. Ruddock says: "As a rule the patient's diet should be restricted for some time to milk and soda water in equal proportions, which is both nourishing and digestible, and may be taken without adding to the patient's discomfort."

Dr. R. J. McClatchey has unbounded faith in "Hydrochloric acid applied with a camels' hair pencil."

Locally the Permanganate of Potash, will be found of great utility.

Prof. Wood in his work on "Practice" says: "I have found nothing so useful as a solution of Sulphate of Zinc, in the proportion of fifteen or twenty grains to the fluid ounce of water, applied twice or three times a day to the ulcer by means of a camels' hair pencil, and continued until the yellowish white exudation is removed, and the surface assumes a reddish hue. With this application I have in no instance failed to effect a cure. It is highly probable that strong solutions of Sulphate of Copper, or Nitrate of Silver, which have been recommended would prove equally effectual."

Any of the mineral acids, diluted with honey or glycerine, and applied with a camel's hair pencil, will be found valuable adjuncts.

Pulverized borax and sugar in equal parts, used locally, has often been of great value.

Glyceroles of Hydrastin used locally has done good service for me.

In desperate cases of parts should be touched daily with a pencil of nitrate of silver.

Calendula, locally, has done good service.

Sulphate of Copper, in substance, applied twice a day, has a fine curative effect.

Glycerine will often prove beneficial, especially if the inside of the cheeks and tongue become dry, with much thirst.

DIARRHEA

Diarrhea, when not occasioned by intestinal tubercles, is treated fully in our text books, but when it is produced by tubercular lesions it is a formidable symptom to contend with, and the physician will often be disappointed with the action of his remedies in this form of diarrhea. Generally it takes place in the last stage of the disease, and cannot well be treated alone, there being so many other prominent symptoms with it. We will, therefore, simply name the most prominent and useful remedies for this form of diarrhea:—

1. Calcarea phosphorica, Phosphorus, Arsenicum, Mercurius, Sulphur, Nitricum acidum, China, Carbo vegetabilis, Phosphoricum acidum, Ferrum and Argentum nitricum.
2. Nux v., Pulsatilla, Colocynth, Terebinth., Baptisia, Collinsonia, Ipecac, Rheum, Antimonium crudum., Podophyllum, Cuprum and Veratrum album.

PRACTICAL EXPEDIENTS

Rest in the recumbent posture. The extremities and the abdomen should be kept warm, the latter by flannel worn over it. Severe gripping pains may often be relieved by flannel heated, or wrung out of hot water, and applied as hot as can be borne. A heated dinner plate applied to the abdomen will often be of much comfort to the patient. If the pains are very severe nothing serves me so well as mustard mixed with the white of an egg. It will not blister in this form, and can be left on for hours. An abdominal compress, six to nine inches wide, and long enough to go round the body, made out to two or three thicknesses of linen, wrung out of cold water and covered with oiled silk, and worn day and night, will often be of great service in controlling the diarrhea. Injections of water often do good. Mucilaginous enemata of flax seed, or flax with a few drops of opium added, often give great relief and quiet rest to the patient when everything else fails. I have used as an injection, a weak solution of the Sulphate of Copper with fine results, also the Sulphate of Zinc. Morphine, internally, in the last stages, when all other means fail us, will be found a great comfort to the patient, and should never be denied.

DIET—During the attack of diarrhea, food should be given sparingly, consisting of gruel, rice, arrow root, sago, or milk. Milk and lime water, as recommended by T.K. Chambers, is often of great value; it alone will frequently arrest the diarrhea, and soda water may occasionally be substituted for the lime water. This alkaline diet should to taken frequently, but in small quantities, Mutton, chicken, pigeon, white fish and game, may generally taken in small quantities. Wholesome ripe fruit may be used in moderation. Mucilaginous drinks such as barley water, gum water, linseed tea, &c. can be used freely; also lemon and orangeade.

PAIN

Pain in the chest, in some becomes so annoying that it calls for special treatment, as a rule pain is taken into consideration as an index to the selection of the remedy, consequently we will omit the remedies and confine our remarks to.

PRACTICAL EXPEDIENTS

In the majority of cases the use of a Belladonna, Rhus tox., or Opium plaster, worn constantly, will be all that is required.

In severe cases, counter irritation, by means of three parts of acetum cantharidis to one of spiritus camphor. This produces slight vesication. but does not cause a permanent sore. Williams uses the tincture of Iodine. An excellent method of relieving pain in phthisis, is by fixing mechanically the entire side with strips of adhesive plaster. The first strip is laid obliquely in the direction of the ribs, the second across the course of the first, the third in the direction of the first, and so on until the entire side is covered. This has often arrested the severest pains of pleurisy.

If the pain comes on very suddenly, and is very severe, I know of nothing better than pure mustard, mixed with the white of an egg; it can be applied readily, every family having more or less of it on hand at all times. Application of heat in the form of poultices, or flannel wrung out of hot water, applied to the painful part, in cases of sudden, intense pain, will be found of much service and comfort to the patient.

Camphorated oil used as a liniment is an excellent remedy to relieve pain.

Dry cupping will often cure pains in the chest as if by magic, and at the same time greatly benefit the breathing.

Our school does not value cupping as it should; in many diseases nothing will help the patient with greater rapidity.

BED SORES

In the last stages of phthisis, the patient is very apt to be greatly troubled with bed sores, from being confined to the bed. They are generally situated about the sacrum and along the spinal column. Internal medication can seldom be resorted to, the patient at the time using other remedies for phthisis; consequently we will have to depend upon practical expedients.

PRACTICAL EXPEDIENTS

The first thing to be done is to lessen the amount of pressure, and this is best obtained by the use of circular air or down cushions, the bed sores should bathed twice a day with a weak solution of Arnica or Calendula, and then dressed with carbolated Calendula cerate.

Dr. Brown-Sequard's treatment has been pronounced successful by those who have tried his method; it consists of applying sponges alternately wetted with hot and cold water to the bed sores, each sponge remaining upon the parts about one minute. Alternately for ten or fifteen minutes, each treatment.

Galvanism has been recommended by Crupel, of St. Petersburgh and Spencer Wells; and Dr. Hammond has greatly extolled its use. He says: "During the last six years I have employed it to a great extent in the treatment of bed sores caused by diseases of the spinal cord, and with scarcely a failure, indeed, I may say, without any failures, except in two cases where deep sinuses had formed which could not be reached by the apparatus. A thin silver plate, no thicker than a sheet of paper, is cut to the exact size and shape of the bed sore, a zinc plate of about the same size is connected with the silver plate by a fine silver or copper wire, six or eight inches in length; the silver plate is then placed in immediate contact with the bed sore, and the zinc plate on some part above, a piece of chamois skin soaked in vinegar intervenes, this must be kept moist or there is little or no action of the battery. Within a few hours there is a perceptible change, and in a day or two the cure is complete in a majority of cases. In a few instances a longer time is required. I have frequently seen bed sores three or four inches in diameter and half an inch deep, heal entirely in forty eight hours. Mr. Spencer Wells states that he has often witnessed large ulcers covered with granulations within twenty-four hours, and completely filled up and cicatrization began in forty eight hours. During his recent visit to this country I informed him of my experience, and he reiterated his opinion that it was the best of all methods for treating ulcers of an indolent character and bed sores."

A dressing of Unguentum Zinci has been used successfully. Glycerine cream has also been found useful.

In very tedious cases, there is nothing so comforting to the patient as a water or air bed.

Preventive treatment is of most importance, which consists of great cleanliness. The skin may be protected by the application of collodion. Soap plaster spread upon wash-leather, amadou, isinglass or felt. The skin should be strengthened by being washed with spirits of wine, either pure, or having two grains of Bichloride of Mercury dissolved in each ounce. Proof spirit, full strength is better than brandy and water, Camphorated spirits and lime water are also useful.

A generous diet is absolutely necessary to build the patient up as fast as possible.

External Application of Chloral— Apropos of this subject, to which we have elsewhere referred, M. Martineau states in *L'Union Pharmaceutique*, that he has derived great advantage from the topical employment of the solutions of chloral. In the bed sores of typhoid fever he uses an aqueous solution of the strength of one per cent., first washing the sore well, and then covering it with lint soaked in this liquid. He says its effect is remarkable; the sloughing, atonic region taking on a healthy aspect, granulating, discharging less and proceeding rapidly towards a cure. When there is offensive suppuration, he used a mixture of chloral and eucalyptus, or carbolic acid lotion—*Medical and Surgical Reporter*.

NUTRITIVE MEAT JELLY

Dr. Anstie, in his lectures on diseases of the nervous system, says when it is necessary to give condensed nutriment in the smallest possible bulk, nothing equals this jelly. "Lean beef fillet 3 pounds; lean veal 3 pounds; lean mutton 3 pounds; cut up into small pieces and put into a saucepan *with no water;* simmer (never boil) by the side of the fire for eight hours; strain the liquid (from a small quantity of tasteless insoluble fibre that remains), and let it jellify into a soft mass. This is an immensely concentrated *meat*, minus very little but the water which has been driven off; a teaspoonful or two of it is a wonderful support, and can be taken every hour with ease."

THE BLOOD CURE

"The practice, which came so rapidly in vogue, of taking for consumption drafts of warm blood the moment when extracted from the calf or ox, has gone into considerable disuse of late, on account of distaste, inconvenience and other reasons. Dr. De Pascale, of Nice, has successfully adopted a substitute in the form of dry powdered blood. The blood of the animal, after being dried in a water bath, is reduced to a very fine powder, and grated through a sieve, and it can thus be taken for any length of time without repugnance, being almost tasteless; can be taken as any common powder, mixed with soups, milk, marmalade, chocolate, or enclosed in a wafer. The quantity of the powder varies according to the patient's age, sex, state of health and digestive power; in general beginning with thirty grains, increasing as circumstances, may dictate."

■■

SPIROMETER

An *instrument* for measuring the capacity of a man's lungs, in cubic inches, in health and disease.

The *spirometer* is the most valuable aid that science has placed in the hands of the physician for detecting diseases of the respiratory organs in their incipiency, and a physician's armamentarium without this instrument is not half filled.

The London *Lancet* says: "This mode of distinguishing consumption at an earlier period than by any other means, has been actually proved."

Dr. Hall, of London, who has made diseases of the lungs a speciality, says the stethoscope is a mere toy compared to the spirometer; his language is: "I consider the stethoscope and plessimeter as mere toys, which do well enough to excite the credulous, but I must confess they never gave me any satisfaction; I never could learn anything by them.

In forming an opinion in a case of consumption the main foundations are:

1st. The condition of the pulse.

2nd. The degree of emaciation.

3rd. The measurement of the lungs (with the spirometer).

4th. The sounds given to the ear when it is laid on the patient's breast, while standing, or back when stooping.

Referring to the spirometer in detecting the early existence of consumption, the London *Lancet* says:-

"It is proven by actual experiment with the spirometer that a man's lungs, found after death to have been tuberculated to the extent of *one inch,* had been by that amount of tubercularization controlled in their action to the extent of more than *forty* cubic inches."

Dr. Hall, in remarking upon this extract, says: "It is very apparent, then that this mode of examination detects the presence of tubercles in their *earliest* formation, which is, in fact, the only time to treat consumption successfully and surely; and when attempted at this early stage, before it is all fixed in the system, the certainty of success in warding off and curing the disease, is as great as that of warding off the cholera, or perfectly curing it, if attempted at the first appearance of the premonitory symptoms; and when cholera is present in the community, every person who has three or more passages from the bowels within twenty four hours, ought to be considered as attacked with the cholera, and should act accordingly. So when a man has tubercles in his lungs to the extent of impairing their functions for a dozen inches, that is when his lungs do not, with other symptoms, hold enough air by a dozen inches, he should consider himself as having consumption, and act accordingly, and with the assurance that in four cases out of five, human life would be saved by it, and as thousands have died with cholera, by hoping they did not have it, or denying they had it, although warned by the usual symptoms at its commencement, until its existence was apparent to the most common observer, rendering a hope of cure impossible, so precisely is it in consumption; people will not take warning by the symptoms in their own persons, which have in thousands of others terminated in certain death, but go on day after day without reason, hoping that the symptoms will go away themselves, and steadily deny that they have the disease until remedy is hopeless. If then, a man should take the alarm as soon as he perceives he is habitually consuming a less amount of air at each act of breathing than he ought to do, whatever may be the cause of it, so, on the other hand, if he finds, on examination, that the lungs contain fully as much air as the system requires, then is it beyond all question that all his lungs are within him in healthful action, and therefore must he perfectly free from consumption, that whatever else may be the matter with him, it most evidently is not phthisis."

Dr. Hall further remarks : "Men are reported to have lived three weeks without food, but without air we cannot live three minutes. The lungs of a full sized man weigh about three pounds, and will hold twelve pints of air; but nine pints are as much as can be inhaled at one full breath, there being always a residuum held in the lungs; that is, all the air that is within them can never be expelled at once. In common, easy breathing, in repose, we inhale one pint. Singers take in from five to seven pints at a single breath. We breathe, in health, about eighteen times in a minute, that is, take in eighteen pints of air in one minute of time, or three thousand gallons in twenty four hours.

"On the other hand, the quantity of blood in a common sized man is twenty pints. The heart beats seventy times a minute, and at each beat throws out four tablespoonsful, that is, two ounces of blood; therefore there passes through the heart and from it to the lungs an amount of blood every twenty four hours equal to two thousand gallons.

"The process of human life, therefore, consists in there meeting together in the lungs, every twenty four hours, two thousand gallons of blood and three thousand gallons of air. Good health requires this absolutely, and cannot be maintained for long with less than the full amount of each; for such are the proportions which nature has ordained and called for. It is easy, therefore, to perceive that in proportion as a person is consuming daily less air than is natural, in such proportion is a decline of health rapid and inevitable. To know, then, how much air a man does habitually consume, is second in importance, in determining his true condition, to no other fact, is a symptom to be noticed and measured in every case of disease, most especially in disease of the lungs, and no man can safely say that the lungs are sound and well, and working fully, until he has ascertained, by actual mathematical measurement, their capacity of action at the time of examination. All else is indefinite, dark conjecture, the great and most satisfactory deduction in all cases being this, that if upon a proper examination, the lungs of any given person are working freely and fully, according to the figures of the case, one thing is incontrovertibly true, demonstrably true, that whatever thousand other things may be the matter with the man, he certainty has nothing like consumption; the announcement and certainty that it is not consumption, brings with it a satisfaction, a gladness of relief, which cannot be measured."

"On the other hand, just in proportion as a person is habitually breathing less air than he ought to do, in such proportion he is falling fast and surely into a fatal disease. This *tendency* to consumption can be usually discovered years in advance of actual occurrence of the disease."

Dr. Flint, in vol.1, of his Physiology of Man, has a most valuable article on the Spirometer, from which I make the following extract:

"*Extreme Breathing Capacity*—By the extreme breathing capacity is meant the volume of air which can be expelled from the lungs by the most forcible expiration, after the most profound inspiration. This has been called by Dr. Hutchinson the *vital capacity,* as signifying "the volume of air which canbe displaced by living movements." It's volume is equal to the sum of the reserve air, the breathing and the complimental air, and represents the extreme capacity of the chest, deducting the residual air. Its physiological interest is due to the fact that it can readily be determined by an appropriate apparatus, the spirometer, and comparisons can thus be made between different individuals, both healthy and diseased. The number of observations on this point by Dr. Hutchinson is enormous, amounting in all to little short of *five thousand.*"

The extreme breathing capacity in health is subject to variations, which has been shown to bear a very close relation to the stature of the individual. Hutchinson commences with the proposition *that in a man of medium height—*(5 *feet,* 8 *inches*), *it is equal to two hundred cubic inches.* He has shown that the extreme breathing capacity is constant in the same individual, and that it is not to be increased by habit or practice, (without there is a diseased condition of the lungs).

The most striking result of the experiments of Dr. Hutchinson, with regard to the modifications of the vital capacity, is that it bears a definite relation to *stature,* without being affected in any very marked degree by *weight,* or the *circumference* of the *chest.* This is especially remarkable, as it is well known that height does not depend so much upon the length of the body, as the length of the lower extremities.

It has been acertained that for every inch in height, between five and six feet, the extreme breathing capacity is increased eight cubic inches. The following table shows the mean results to the immense number of observations on which this conclusion is based:

Progression of the Vital Capacity Volume with the Stature.

Height.	Series from observations on 1,012 cases.	Series from observations on 1923 cases.	Series in arithmetical progression.
	First result.	*Second result.*	
5 feet 0 inches, 5 " 2 " } 5 feet 1 inch...	175.0	176.0	174.0
5 " 2 ", 5 " 4 " } 5 feet 3 inch.....	188.5	191.0	190.0
5 " 4 ", 5 " 6 " } 5 feet 5 inch.....	206.0	206.0	206.0
5 " 6 ", 5 " 8 " } 5 feet 7 inch.....	222.0	228.0	222.0
5 " 8 ", 5 " 10 " } 5 feet 9 inch.....	237.0	246.0	238.0
5 " 10 ", 6 " 0 " } 5 feet 11 inch...	254.0	258.0	254.0
Mean of all heights............	214.0	217.0	214.0

Age has an influence, though less marked than stature, upon the extreme breathing capacity. As the result of 4,800 observations (males), it was ascertained that the volume increases with age up to the thirtieth year, and progressively decreases, with tolerable regularity, from the thirtieth to the sixtieth year.

These figures, though necessarily subject to certain individual variations, may be taken as the basis for examinations of the extreme breathing capacity in disease, which frequently gives important information. Of course, the breathing capacity is modified by an abnormal condition which interferes with the mobility of the thorax, or the dilatability of the lungs. Of all diseased conditions, phthisis pulmonalis is the most interesting in this connection. With regard to the significance of the variations in this disease. Dr. Hutchinson has arrived at the following conclusions:

"It has been found that ten cubic inches below the due quantity, *i.e.*, 220 instead of 230 cubic inches, need not excite alarm, but there is a point of deficiency in the breathing volume, at which it is difficult to say whether it is merely one of those physiological differences dependent on a certain irregularity in all such observations, or deficiency indicative of disease. A deficiency of sixteen per cent. is suspicious. A man below fifty five years of age, breathing 193 cubic inches instead of 230 cubic inches, unless he is excessively fat, is probably the subject of disease.

"In phthisis pulmonalis the deficiency may amount to 90 per cent., and yet life be maintained. The vital capacity volume is likewise a measure of improvement. A phthisical patient may improve so as to gain 40 upon 220 cubic inches."

"Herbst has shown that the extreme breathing capacity is diminished by obesity; that it is proportionally less in females than in males and in children than in adult."

Dr. Hall gives us a fine illustration of the practical workings of the *spirometer* on page 167 of his work on "Bronchitis and Kindred Diseases", by giving twelve fatal cases of phthisis :

Case 1. Had lost five-tenths of her lung measurement, and died in twelve days.
Case 2. Had lost five-tenths, and died in eight months.
Case 3. Had lost four-tenths, and died in two months.
Case 4. Had lost two-tenths, and died in six months.
Case 5. Had lost four-tenths, and died in two weeks.
Case 6. Had lost six-tenths, and died in two weeks.
Case 7. Had lost four-tenths, and died in four months.

Case 8. Had lost three-tenths, and died in three months.
Case 9. Had lost three-tenths, and died in four months.
Case 10. Had lost three-tenths, and died in three months.
Case 11. Had lost three-tenths, and died in two months.
Case 12. Had lost three-tenths, and died in three months.

I have given twelve consecutively fatal, measured cases, occurring during twelve consecutive months, known to have died from direct observation, by which it will be seen that persons having consumptive symptoms, and who had lost the use of three-tenths of the lungs or more, died in four months, three only having lived longer.

It will be seen that No. 2 with a loss of five-tenths, which is one-half, lived eight months, while No. 4 with a loss of two-tenths or one-fifth only, lived only two weeks; this difference arises from the fact that the loss of measurement, in all cases, arises from two causes, first, the loss of lung substance; second, the loss of lung function only; the greater the loss of lung substance, the sooner the patient dies, but *vice versa,* when the greater portion of the loss is not because the lungs have decayed away, but because they work imperfectly from being filled up with matter or mucus, or tubercles, or from mere inaction. Auscultation must decide what proportions of the deficit is attributable to the respective causes, and from that, we must judge the probable time of termination. When the deficiency is large, and auscultation shows no decay, no actual loss of lung substance, there is an encouraging ground for restoration, if prompt attention is given to treatment."

These cases are followed by a few cases that recovered, showing the increase of lung measurement as health was restored:

Case 1, Nov. 24. Deficiency from full measurement, one-tenth; March 11th, dismissed cured, with full measuremens, and four years after remained well.

Case 2, Dec. 18. Deficiency, two-tenths; Jan. 14, fully restored, and known to be in good health for four years, with full measurement.

Case 3, Dec. 18. Deficiency, three-tenths; April 17, deficiency nearly restored, and enjoyed good health for three years.

Case 4, Dec. 8. Deficiency, three-tenths; pulse 120; March 22nd, restored; pulse, 72.

The doctor gives several more cases, but I have given enough to illustrate my point; he closes by saying that, "the prominent parts to be noticed in the twelve cases given are:

1. That when there is but a small deficiency in the measurement of the lungs, it is uniformly restored, by appropriate means, persevered in.
2. That when such deficiency is made up, the system returns to good health.

And the great practical lesson to be derived from the two classes of cases is:

That inasmuch as when the deficiency is large, persons usually die within half a year.

That when, on the other hand, the deficiency is small, health is generally regained in a reasonable time.

Spirometry is a mathematical measurement designated by figures, which answers to a certain set of conditions.

The amount of air capable of being expired from a man's lungs is accurately measured to a single cubic inch, or half inch. Different persons require a different amount of air, but these are regulated by nature herself, who modifies them by certain fixed proportions.

Sex.	Age.	Breath.	Pulse.	Height.	Weight.	Capacity.
Male	40	17	68	6 feet	140	262 cubic in.

These seven correspondents occurring in one man, are *unfailing* indications of the full healthful condition of the lungs, and when the pulse and breathing are steadily over these, and the lung capacity is under in such a man for a month or two, *then the foundations of consumption are being made,* and infallibly 50 as far as my experience has gone. But these deviations are seldom alone. Notes of alarm are sounded in other parts of the empire of life."

Females measure less than males, varying from ten to fifteen per cent. The following table will make it more practical:

Height 4 feet 8 inches, male capacity, 134, female capacity, 96 cubic in.
,,	4	,,	9	,,	,,	,,	142	,,	,,	104	,,	,,
,,	4	,,	10	,,	,,	,,	150	,,	,,	112	,,	,,
,,	4	,,	11	,,	,,	,,	158	,,	,,	120	,,	,,
,,	5	,,	0	,,	,,	,,	166	,,	,,	128	,,	,,
,,	5	,,	1	,,	,,	,,	174	,,	,,	136	,,	,,
,,	5	,,	2	,,	,,	,,	182	,,	,,	144	,,	,,
,,	5	,,	3	,,	,,	,,	190	,,	,,	152	,,	,,
,,	5	,,	4	,,	,,	,,	198	,,	,,	160	,,	,,
,,	5	,,	5	,,	,,	,,	206	,,	,,	168	,,	,,
,,	5	,,	6	,,	,,	,,	214	,,	,,	176	,,	,,
,,	5	,,	7	,,	,,	,,	222	,,	,,	184	,,	,,
,,	5	,,	8	,,	,,	,,	230	,,	,,	192	,,	,,
,,	5	,,	9	,,	,,	,,	238	,,	,,	200	,,	,,
,,	6	,,	10	,,	,,	,,	246	,,	,,	208	,,	,,
,,	5	,,	11	,,	,,	,,	254	,,	,,	216	,,	,,
,,	6	,,	0	,,	,,	,,	262	,,	,,	224	,,	,,

"Some persons six feet in height will exhibit a lung capacity of 300 cubic inches, and others of the same height may measure no more than 224 inches, and yet enjoy good health; and so in proportion through the entire table. With this standard in view, the intelligent physician, with a little practice, will soon be able to determine whether the lungs are diseased or not, and the extent of the same." The above table is the average measurement in five thousand cases, and is near enough for all practical purposes. Trained singers in good health will go over the average measurement, and it is a well established fact that they seldom die with pulmonary consumption, showing the great utility of deep, full breathing. The practice of elocution, gymnastics, and the constant use of breathing tubes, with the spirometer, *cannot be urged too strongly* upon those that are *predisposed to pulmonary consumption.* Phthisical patients should be *constantly* urged to get into the habit of *deep, full* breathing. Full, deep breathing exercises every part of the lungs, while feeble, ordinary breathing, only exercises the lower lobes, leaving the upper lobes dormant, which explains why tubercles always commence in the upper lobes; every muscle and tissue that is not used, becomes feeble, and is then the centre or focus for any disease the system may be predisposed to.

Professor Juergensen, in the Cyclopædia of the Practice of Medicine, Vol. V., page 487, speaking of lung capacity in those predisposed to phthisis, mentions a fact well worth remembering; he says: "If the chest were filled with 600 cen. of solid matter, especially if the latter were concentrated in the upper parts of the lungs, percussion would, doubtlessly, show the fact; and even if, in all these cases, we suppose that the first ribs are immovable, the deficit would be too great. The only explanation left is, that the deficit is due to feebleness of the respiratory muscles. What is known as the *paralytic thorax* seems to be traceable to this factor, *loss of muscular power*. The slender neck, the prominent clavicles, the broad, depressed, intercostal spaces, and the scapulæ projecting like wings show that the principal respiratory muscles have been atrophied. The main burden of respiration is therefore thrown upon the diaphragm in the very years when there should be a due co-operation on the part of the other muscles."

This explains why those predisposed to phthisis have less lung capacity than those that do not have this predisposition, and should be taken into consideration in spirometry.

I have found that the loss of a night's sleep, habitual drinks of intoxicating liquors, even ever so slight if indulged in daily, greatly diminishes the lung capacity. Also a full stomach. The spirometer should not be used directly after eating.

Heretofore the *spirometer* has not been utilized by the mass of practicing physicians, for the simple reason *all* that have been put into the market have been so large and bungling, that their use had to be confined to the office, and then the use of one took up so much valuable time that the practitioner could not afford to use it. To illustrate it more fully, I will take Dr. G. W. Brown's valuable spirometer, in all probability as good an instrument as can be found in the market. To take it down, adjust it, fill it with water (it takes several gallons), use it, take it apart again, wipe it dry to keep it from rust, about one hour is consumed. This hour to the physician is worth from two to five dollars, and he cannot charge that much for his services, consequently he cannot afford to use it, and then if his patient has to be visited at his residence, the spirometer cannot be used at all, because of the great trouble a transporting it from house to house.

To get the spirometer in a small enough compass, so as to be carried constantly in the physician's pocket, has been a source of constant study to me for the last two years, and it gives me great pleasure in being able to announce to the profession that I have succeeded in producing an instrument whose *action* is *perfect* as a *thermometer*, can be carried in the pocket, taken out and used, and replaced in the pocket in two minutes, and only costs a mere trifle, compared to those now in use, at once utilizing this greatest of all instruments for diseases of the lungs.